D0207104

What others are saying

Critical Conditions
The Essential Hospital Guide
to Get Your Loved One Out Alive

"Martine has accomplished what scores of nurses have talked about for years. She has collected crucial helpful hints and organized them together in an easy to understand format, for family members who have a loved one in the hospital. When lay people enter this 'foreign country' of hospitals and rehab facilities, the language, practices, strange sounds and equipment are often intimidating. This book is their survival guide. Martine's mantra: 'to support the best possible medical care for your loved one,' is really what every member of the health care team is striving for. Many instances of a breakdown in communication or trust between the health care team and the patient or family can be avoided by using this tool. Before I finished reading it, I had made a list of friends who need a copy. This book belongs in the gift shop of every hospital." **JACKIE KOOB, RN, BSN, STANTON, CA**

"They should pass out this book to all families who have loved ones in hospitals." **ROBERT ADAIR, MD, SANTA MONICA, CA**

"*Critical Conditions* is a most comprehensive guidebook for the individual who has a loved one in the hospital. It provides the do's and don'ts for the family.

"Ms. Ehrenclou is to be complimented on having written a practical and informative book."

HOWARD S. TRAISMAN, MD, EMERITUS PROFESSOR OF PEDIATRICS, NORTHWESTERN UNIVERSITY, FEINBERG SCHOOL OF MEDICINE AND EMERITUS ATTENDING ENDOCRINOLOGIST, CHILDREN'S MEMORIAL HOSPITAL, CHICAGO, IL

"Health care is exceedingly complex and the entire industry is undergoing a significant transition of learning how to further improve the processes of care so that patients are consistently receiving safer and higher quality care in all settings. This type of transition takes time, however, so patients and their families must take the important steps of learning how to ensure optimal care for themselves by collaborating with the professionals who are providing their care. This book is well-written and organized with an intuitive layout such that patients and their families will benefit from its use for a single short-term hospital stay—as well as for long-term multiple hospital stays. A great patient and family resource."   **PETER B. ANGOOD MD, FRCS, FACS, FCCM**
VICE-PRESIDENT & CHIEF PATIENT SAFETY OFFICER
THE JOINT COMMISSION, CHICAGO, IL

"*Critical Conditions* provides the 411 on a 911 situation. This book is a practical resource that teaches HOW and WHY to be a champion, an observer, a voice for our hospitalized loved ones; a personal reference that feels like an experienced friend; AND a step-by-step roadmap that guides readers from Admitting, past the confusion of hospitalization, through the fears, along the path of safe and efficient care, and finally to Discharge. Readers will learn how collaborative communication between physicians, nurses, hospital staff, and family members and their loved ones can only enhance the quality, experience, and outcome for our most vulnerable health care recipients.

"*Critical Conditions* will be equally appropriate for the medical school or college classroom, in a suitcase bound for the hospital, at the admitting office or emergency room, on a bed stand, and in the hands of every patient advocate."   **LUCY HU BRUTTOMESSO, MD, LOS ANGELES, CA**

"As an RN who has also had critically ill loved ones in the hospital, I feel that this book is an important and empowering tool. It covers the process from beginning to end and enables the reader to navigate the system while still being supportive of the healthcare community."

LESLIE PLATT, RN, LAKEWOOD, CA

"You are the best advocate for your loved one. This book will help guide you through the ins and outs of the hospital system. It gives great guidance on how to be an advocate. The most important thing when you are in the hospital is to have someone be your voice."

SHEILA HELLER, RN, BSN, ARLINGTON, VA

"This book offers invaluable information on the intricacies of hospitalizations. It is written for the public as well as being a refresher for the medical professional, now on the 'other side of the bed.' When someone you love is hospitalized, you will have another full-time job. This book will make that job easier."

PHYLLIS SETLEN, RN, BALTIMORE, MD

"This is a guide or handbook for persons with loved ones in the hospital. It describes, in encyclopedic fashion, how to cope with this foreign medical and technological world. Hospitalization is confusing for the patient, and they may be unaware or unable to function for themselves because of their illness or injury. Now enter the advocate, e.g., the spouse, relative, friend, etc., who also may be confused. However, this book provides a valuable step-by-step guide for maneuvering and negotiating the treacherous maze of hospitalization. It is not everything for everyone, but it does have something for everyone who has a loved one in the hospital. Its comprehensive coverage of topics provides valuable instruction and advice presented in easy to understand lay terms."

PERRY A. HENDERSON, MD, PROFESSOR EMERITUS,
DEPARTMENT OF OBSTETRICS AND GYNECOLOGY,
UNIVERSITY OF WISCONSIN MEDICAL SCHOOL, MADISON, WI

"I wish I'd had your book when my mom was in the hospital. Maybe it would have helped save her life."

B. MARCUS, FAMILY MEMBER, LOS ANGELES, CA

"This book will be a useful tool for understanding and keeping track of vital information throughout the hospitalization. It will prove especially helpful to those navigating this experience for the first time."

AMY EDEN, RN, BSN, LNC, CA

"This book exceeds my expectations. I wish I'd had it for myself and my family years ago. *Critical Conditions* will be in hand if any of us are hospitalized. This book is number one for our family and friends."

MIA VLOET, RN, NEWPORT BEACH, CA

"*Critical Conditions* is a great tool for navigating the hospital system. It provides simple and helpful steps that family members and patients themselves can follow."

MEREDITH SINGER, RN, MSN, BALTIMORE, MD

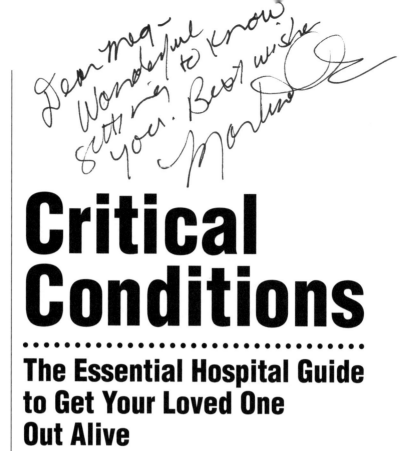

Critical
Conditions

The Essential Hospital Guide to Get Your Loved One Out Alive

Martine Ehrenclou, M.A.

LEMON
GROVE
PRESS

Critical Conditions:
The Essential Hospital Guide to Get Your Loved One Out Alive

By Martine Ehrenclou, MA

Lemon Grove Press, LLC
1223 Wilshire Blvd.
Suite 1750
Santa Monica, CA 90403-5400

Fax: (310) 451-1968
info@criticalconditions.com
www.criticalconditions.com

Copyright © 2008 by Martine Ehrenclou.

All rights reserved. Only the Quick Reference Guide and Daily Progress Notes may be photocopied for personal use. No other part of this book may be reproduced or transmitted in any form or by any means, electronic or mechanical, including photocopying, recording, and/or any information storage and retrieval system, without written permission from the author.

ISBN: 978-0-9815240-0-9
Library of Congress Control Number: 2008902405

First Edition: Printed in the United States of America
0 9 8 7 6 5 4 3 2 1

Cover Design
George Foster

Interior Design & Layout
Sue Knopf, Graffolio

For my mom and Martha

Contents

Note to the Reader

The purpose of this book is to inform and motivate readers by providing an overview of what is involved in acting as advocate for a hospitalized family member and thereby attempting to maximize the care of their loved one. It is not meant to encourage readers to contradict, disregard, interrupt, interfere with, or supersede any medical advice or medical care that is provided by medical professionals in the hospital setting.

This book is not all-inclusive and does not substitute for consultation with appropriate professionals. Although the book encourages increased understanding about being a patient's advocate, all readers are strongly encouraged to consult with experienced health-care practitioners and other professionals. This book is sold with the understanding that the publisher and author are not engaged in rendering medical, legal, financial, or other professional services. If any such expert assistance is required, the services of a competent professional should be sought.

Every effort has been made to make this book as complete and accurate as possible based on the information available at the time of publication. However, there may be mistakes, both typographical and in content, and the accuracy of the contents may change over time. Therefore, this text should be used only as a general guide and not the ultimate source of information about overseeing and supporting medical care for one's hospitalized loved one.

This book is sold without warranties or guarantees of any kind. The author and publisher shall have neither liability nor responsibility to any person or entity with respect to any loss or damage caused or alleged to have been caused, directly or indirectly, by the information in this book.

The author and publisher express their appreciation to individuals who have participated in the preparation of this book and consented to the use of material provided by them. However, no sponsorship or affiliation with, or endorsement by, any such individuals is claimed or suggested.

In some instances, the names and other identifying characteristics of individuals and institutions have been withheld or changed to preserve confidentiality. Any similarity between a fictionalized individual or institution and real individuals and institutions is purely coincidental.

Foreword

THE ETHICAL CODE, which every physician and every nurse you will encounter in a hospital has sworn to uphold, promises that they will do good, avoid harm, treat justly and accept the patient's wishes as the ultimate authority. They do try, for the most part.

But hospitals today are institutions struggling to survive in an environment where authority is in the hands of insurance companies rather than patients and their families. Rapid advancement in technology makes ever more expensive treatments in wide demand. Nurses are more expensive and harder to find and retain. Doctors treating patients in hospitals are more likely to be specialists, whose concerns seem more directed toward a tumor or organ system rather than toward a human being. Communication may sound like a foreign language to the uninitiated. The pace of the staff is usually somewhere between harried and frenetic. Patients are sometimes referred to as "517B" or "the breast cancer in 2112." Serious infections, which are often treated in hospitals, are inadvertently spread from one patient to another.

All of these factors are serious impediments to the compassionate care and the good outcome we all desire when hospitalization is necessary. Ms. Ehrenclou has constructed a practical guide for the patient advocate who commits to active involvement in his or her loved one's hospitalization. There are no easy answers, but there are plenty of suggestions for navigating a system which is, after all, a human institution, one where human factors can and do determine how a person who is also a patient will be perceived and cared for.

Critical Conditions: The Essential Hospital Guide to Get Your Loved One Out Alive will help patient advocates to understand, negotiate and amend the treatment process and decrease errors. Being an active part of the hospital experience benefits both patients and hospital staff, as it encompasses a truly "patient-focused" approach.

Karen Blanchard, MD
Santa Monica, California
June 2008

Acknowledgments

THERE ARE SO MANY PEOPLE to thank who contributed to and supported this book. To my husband, Jamie, for his loving support and encouragement throughout this entire process. To my daughter, Lucy, and my stepson, Logan, for their love, patience, and encouragement. To Rachel Ballon, for her untiring enthusiasm, support, and encouragement—you believed in this from the beginning—thank you. To the team of people who helped me wrangle this book to completion, including the wonderful nurses and physicians whom I interviewed and who offered such valuable insights. To the family members who were willing to share their stories. Thank you all from the bottom of my heart.

Many, many thanks to Sarah Gallwey; Fran Ginsberg; Loren Alison; Victoria Bloch; Judy Quay; W. Knox Richardson; Arlyn Augarten; Annika Baker; Nancy Stark; Robin Iezman; Barbara Marcus; Debbie Berman; Susan Leverton; Ann Fox; Jeanne Weiner; Rob Small; Hank Antosz; Gail Uellendahl; Jasmine Love; Marc Ballon; John Ballon; Karen McChrystal; Karen Blanchard, MD; Robert Adair, MD; Howard S. Traisman, MD; Perry A. Henderson, MD; Lucy Hu Bruttomesso, MD; Peter Angood, MD; David Wellisch, PhD; Phyllis Setlen, RN; Leslie Platt, RN; Jackie Koob, RN; Amy Eden, RN; Mia Vloet, RN; Meredith Singer, RN; Cheryl Nguyen, RN; Sheila Heller, RN; Cheri Adrian, PhD; Jonathan Kirsch; Chuck Wagner; Andrea Stein, MD; Carter Dillman, MD; Carol Pfannkuche; Natalie Soloway; and Ellen Riches.

Much appreciation to Kristin Langenfeld, Karen McChrystal, Sue Knopf, and Melissa Browne for editing and proofreading the manuscript; and to Rachel Rice for creating the index.

Introduction

They should pass this book out to all families who have loved ones in hospitals.

ROBERT ADAIR, MD, SANTA MONICA, CA

THE ONLY TIME I'D EVER SPENT in a hospital was when I gave birth to our daughter. So I was completely unprepared five years later when I got a call that my mother was in the ICU in a hospital in Colorado. I was on the next plane from Los Angeles.

My mother's care was in the hands of doctors and nurses I'd never met, and I didn't know the first thing about hospitals, procedures, treatments, or medications. I certainly didn't understand my role in her care.

The hospital itself was like a walk on the moon. Everything about it was completely unfamiliar. I didn't understand how the hospital system worked, couldn't comprehend medical language, wasn't knowledgeable about how to sift through differing opinions from doctors and nurses, and was frustrated by not being able to reach any of the doctors directly.

I was told my mom had acute pancreatitis. When I asked the nurse what that was, she offered a cryptic definition and suggested I speak with my mother's internist. I asked her how to reach him. She offered the most valuable piece of information that I used not only with my

1

mother's hospitalization but with other close family members who were hospitalized soon after.

She said, "Be here during doctors' rounds first thing in the morning. Be here by 8 AM and just wait. You will be able to meet the doctors face-to-face, ask them questions and find out what is planned for your mother's treatment."

That was the beginning of my education on hospitals.

Had I known what I know now, I would not have left everything up to the medical staff. Physicians and nurses are the experts, and they certainly know what they are doing, but because my mother's condition fluctuated so much, I was in a constant state of reacting to the drastic declines in her physical condition and couldn't think straight.

Because I took a passive role in her care and left everything up to the doctors and nurses, I simply accepted everything they told me at face value. I never questioned a possible medication interaction or allergy, never questioned the onset of pneumonia two months into her hospital stay, and never asked why she contracted a severe staph infection that required heavy doses of several different antibiotics. Not that those two diseases could have been eradicated, but if I had known what I know now, I could have implemented several strategies to help prevent them.

I didn't question my mom's rapid decline when she was moved to a step-down unit after a procedure. Again, I panicked and couldn't think straight. All I cared about was her recovery. What I wasn't aware of then is that the nurse-to-patient ratio fell dramatically on that floor, meaning there were fewer nurses to care for patients. I assumed she was receiving the same quality of care as in the ICU. Not so. What I've learned is that nurses on other floors can be so overwhelmed by the number of patients they care for and by the lack of support nursing staff, that they are juggling patient overload with massive paperwork.

When my mother was in pain, I couldn't understand why the nurses didn't respond to the call button.

I do now.

And now I understand how I could have intervened.

After her drastic decline in the step-down unit, my mother was readmitted to the ICU and put on full life support, which included a trach tube and ventilator, intravenous food, and monitors for her heart, oxygen level, and urine output.

I cannot put into words the heartbreak I felt witnessing her suffering. And to make matters worse, I felt helpless to do anything about it other than to put cold washcloths on her forehead, massage her hands, brush her hair, and feed her ice chips. Because I held the belief that doctors and nurses were superhuman and were handling everything with the ultimate precision of care, I put full faith in their expertise. When I asked about her health decline, they all said it was due to the nature of her disease.

When my mom was placed on full life support her condition worsened. This was the time when her internist took a vacation and another internist showed up, one who had never seen my mother before. That was mind-numbing in itself considering how ill she was. But then I didn't know what I know now. If I had, I would have initiated an in-depth conversation with the new internist about her condition, described what had been tried, and then would have asked him what he planned to do. I would have told him about who my mom was as a human being, so she wouldn't have been regarded as just another patient under his care for a mere two weeks.

Looking back, there were plenty of mistakes along the way, some of which I might have been able to prevent had I been aware that medical errors in hospitals do happen with alarming frequency. But at the time, all I was concerned with were the dramatic setbacks to her recovery after new medications were introduced, a procedure that failed, an unrelenting staph infection, respiratory treatments that left her gagging and gasping for breath, hospital pneumonia, hospital psychosis, and a host of other harrowing incidents.

I never thought to ask about a correlation of my mother's condition to problems with her medical care. I simply sat by, watched, and comforted her as best as I could. I couldn't pinpoint errors because I wasn't aware of their possibility. I didn't know what to watch for. Most of those five months she spent in the hospital were a blur to me.

My mother was incapable of caring for herself, of advocating for herself, or of calling for help when she needed it. I never would have left her alone when I needed to travel back to California had I known that I could have hired a private duty nurse or sitter to fill in for me. I shudder to think of what might have happened in that hospital when I was gone.

Knowing what I do now, I would have carefully monitored her medications and treatments, and I would have asked thorough questions about her decline. I would have researched her disease and maybe even considered transferring her to a larger, metropolitan hospital that might have had more experienced specialists for her disease.

But I didn't know. I wasn't aware of all the options.

Eight months after my mother's death, my godmother, Martha, fell ill. At this point I was at least a little more hospital savvy. She and I were very close, and she called me when she was short of breath and needed to be driven to the hospital. I took her to the ER in two different hospitals a dozen times over the next year and a half because of congestive heart failure, renal failure (which wasn't diagnosed until several months into her last hospital stay), and complications due to her diabetes.

Her last hospital stay was for seven months. I was determined to educate myself this time on all aspects of the hospital system and her care. I eventually learned how to advocate for her. But that wasn't until she went into insulin shock twice in the hospital and almost died, was subjected to a medication error that put her into a near coma for three days and was misdiagnosed with a stroke, developed a bedsore the size of a football because the nurses weren't turning her often enough, was subjected to roommates with dementia who screamed at her in the middle of the night, endured a nurse's abusive treatment, was given a diet filled with sugar, and was given inadequate amounts of insulin.

She ended up wasting away after losing fifty pounds and was put on full life support with a trach tube and ventilator, intravenous food, oxygen, and monitors that calculated her heartbeat, oxygen level, and urine output. Like my mother, Martha ended up not able to get out of bed, not able to speak, and not able to press the nurse's button if she was in need.

By the time she died, she had been subjected to neglect, misdiagnosis, medication allergies, medication errors, and inappropriate care. Worst of all, she suffered needlessly, miserably.

I was determined after these two experiences to find out if my mother's and godmother's experiences were the norm.

I found out that in fact they were. Among the fifty families I interviewed, some with extreme cases like my family members, others with less extreme cases, all expressed immense concern over what had happened to their hospitalized loved ones. Some cited belief in fatal medical mistakes. Others talked about total neglect. All expressed complete confusion about the hospital system and how it is run. Each and every family member reported feeling helpless.

One woman, Barb, whom I interviewed, still believes, five years later, that the hospital killed her mother. She stated that her mother went into the hospital healthy and alert for a simple procedure and ended up having a fatal heart attack on the operating table. She is convinced that something went wrong during the procedure. But no medical professional provided her with answers. So she is left with the feeling that maybe she should have done something to be more involved. Like me, she had full faith in the physicians and nurses. She said, "I wish I'd had your book when my mom was in the hospital. Maybe it would have helped save her life."

I've heard dozens of similar stories from family members who had loved ones go into the hospital and for reasons unknown to them, never came out. They either developed hospital pneumonia, or something went wrong with a procedure, or they contracted a series of hospital diseases and in the end, couldn't fight them off.

I decided that I had to find out directly from registered nurses and doctors about what was happening in hospitals and what family members could do to help their hospitalized loved ones. All of the more than eighty-five hospital registered nurses, dozens of physicians, hospital social workers, physician assistants, and other hospital staff I interviewed said the same thing:

> *You must have someone, a family member, in the hospital*
> *with the patient at all times. Hospital care is in crisis.*

This book is for anyone who has a loved one in the hospital. It is particularly useful for those whose loved ones are seriously ill or have multiple medical conditions and for those whose loved ones have suffered a medical error or have taken a turn for the worse.

This book will teach you how to be an effective and caring advocate for your loved one. It will teach you how to support the nurses and physicians so they can do the job they truly want to do, but can't because of the drastic nursing shortage, the demands on doctors to see too many patients in too little time, and the financial duress hospitals are now under. Everyone in the medical profession is trying to do the best job they can.

There is something you can do to help. This book will teach you how.

You will learn how to get more attention for your loved one, how to communicate effectively with doctors and nurses, and how to actually reach them. With the help of this book, you will more easily sift through differing diagnoses and opposing opinions about the status of your loved one. You will be more prepared to decide when to bring in a second opinion, or even a third.

Each chapter is based on a series of "Steps" to guide you, complete with sample questions and space for checklists and notes. You may think you'll remember every detail of your conversations with your loved one's doctors and nurses, but I can almost promise you, you won't. Stress plays amazing tricks with one's memory. *Write everything down in this book.* There is space at the end of every chapter to take quick notes on that chapter's material. You will also need to write all essential information in the Quick Reference Guide at the back of the book. The back-of-the-book Guide will serve as a convenient reference not only for you, but also for all the other members of your Family Advocate Team.

Use this book as a handbook, a diary of patient progress, of procedures, medications, tests, and conversations. *Take notes. Take notes. Take notes.*

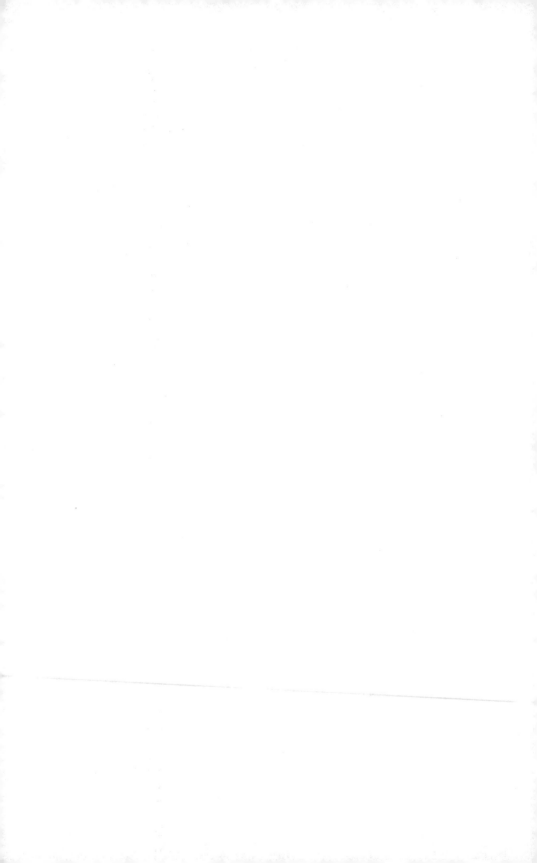

CHAPTER 1

You Could Save a Life

A patient shouldn't be expected to look out for him or herself while in the hospital; a family member should be the patient's strongest ally/friend/protector.

ANONYMOUS MD, ST. VINCENT'S HOSPITAL, NY

IF YOUR LOVED ONE IS IN THE HOSPITAL experiencing a medical crisis or undergoing surgery or some form of treatment for a severe illness, you are most likely stressed. You are probably worried about their condition and may be feeling helpless. The hospital may be completely unfamiliar to you. Hospitals aren't fun places to be. You may not even want to be there. No one wants to be there, including your loved one, who is being poked and prodded, fed unappetizing food and put through stress not just by procedures, operations, or treatments, but simply by being a patient in the hospital. Think of them when you read this book.

Your natural instinct might be to surrender control to the hospital staff because you believe that they know what they are doing.

And they do.

But the first thing you must be aware of is that no matter how skilled and committed the nurses and physicians are in your loved one's case, most cannot overcome patient overload. That translates to a higher probability of medical error.

There is something you can do.

A nationwide, drastic nursing shortage means fewer nurses to tend to your loved one. Even if there is a nurse-to-patient ratio law in your state (in California, it's 1:5), in all likelihood the hospital has had to cut back on support staff so it has the financial ability to hire the required number of registered nurses. In many cases, your hospital has had to cut certified nursing assistants (CNAs), licensed vocational nurses (LVNs), nurse's aides, respiratory therapists, lab technicians, etc. That means the registered nurses are now not only doing their own jobs, but the jobs of the staff who have been cut.

There is something you can do.

Because hospitals are now restricting admissions to patients who need care the most, patients are now sicker than ever before. Translation? Doctors and nurses are caring for patients who need more of their attention.

There are now more older patients because of the baby boomer generation. This increases the number of patients with multiple medical issues, who are at risk of falling out of bed and breaking bones or contracting a hospital disease that could kill them. Nurses have to pay even more attention to this patient population.

In addition, the spread of infectious diseases (pneumonia, MRSA, etc.) has increased to shocking proportions. That means there's even more for nurses and doctors to monitor and keep track of.

To compound the above issues, doctors are required by insurance companies to see more patients in less time. Their time is divided among patients they see in their offices, in hospitals, and in surgeries. This is part of the reason that the role of physician's assistant is becoming so popular. Doctors just can't keep up.

Hospitals are now inundated with patients who don't have insurance and who don't pay their bills. Half of the nation's emergency departments are at or over capacity. Hospitals continue to face significant increases in the costs of pharmaceuticals and other supplies and face workforce shortages that are affecting patient care.

There is something you can do.

Nurses and doctors are overworked and overwhelmed. Most claim they cannot do the job they aspire to. Many hospitals are not able to provide the precision of care necessary to avoid the number of preventable, fatal, medical errors that occur with their patients, many of which are highly publicized.

This is where you come in.

A loved one who is in pain or sick cannot possibly be their own advocate. They cannot oversee their own care. Try to imagine being really sick with the flu or being heavily medicated for pain and trying to talk about your medical issues with nurses and doctors.

It's practically impossible.

It is your job as a family member to do this for the patient. You must oversee and support medical care—in essence, be a sentinel. This means monitoring daily patient progress, talking in person with doctors and nurses, tracking results of procedures and medications, taking steps to help prevent the spread of hospital communicable diseases, medical errors and falls, and monitoring the effectiveness of the care provided.

Remember, your loved one's hospital stay is time limited. You won't be doing this forever, but your efforts now could save a life.

No medical professional in the hospital is purposely avoiding your loved one, purposely being negligent, or intentionally causing errors. Nurses and doctors are all doing the best jobs they can. But what you will learn to do as a result of reading this book is to reduce the chances of your loved one becoming a statistic.

Your role is to support the medical care being provided. In no way will you be taking charge of it, displacing nurses or doctors, or superseding the medical interventions. You will simply be the watchdog and a support for the medical professionals caring for your loved one.

Almost every doctor and nurse I interviewed said this: "Patients recover faster when the family is involved."

The unfortunate reality is this:

- The Fifth Annual HealthGrades Patient Safety in American Hospitals Study, 2008, found that patient safety incidents resulted in 238,337 potentially preventable deaths during 2004 through 2006. HealthGrades previously estimated that within the entire population, not just Medicare patients, there were 575,000 preventable deaths caused by medical errors over three years.

- CBS News (Jan. 17, 2003): "American hospitals are in serious crisis, from large numbers of uninsured patients to spiraling costs, from outlandishly expensive prescription drugs to a severe and dangerous shortage of nurses."

- *Time* (May 1, 2006) reported in its cover story, "What Doctors Hate About Hospitals," that "Until proper safeguards are built into the system, what a patient needs most, many doctors agree, is a sentinel—someone to take notice, to be an advocate, ask questions."

Family's Story

Susan's husband suffered a major heart attack. Manni had surgery to insert a stent. Right after his surgery, he was put in a hospital room in the cardiac wing. An oxygen mask was placed on his face. He said to his wife that there was no oxygen coming through. Susan asked the primary nurse about this, and the nurse explained that the oxygen was a light dose.

Several hours later, Manni again said that no oxygen was coming through the mask. Susan traced the oxygen line and was shocked to find that the oxygen line was not even plugged into the wall. It was tucked behind Manni's pillow.

Imagine if Susan hadn't been there, and her husband had been in dire need of oxygen.

- A recent study (Feb. 2006) done by US Pharmacopoeia and published by Reuters reported 38,000 medication mistakes within one year in a sample of 56 hospital ICUs nationwide.

- ABC News (Oct. 23, 2005), citing the Centers for Disease Control and Prevention, reported that as many as 100,000 people die in this country each year from infections they get in the hospital.

- *The New England Journal of Medicine* (May 30, 2002) reported that when there are too few registered nurses at bedsides, patients are significantly more likely to suffer serious complications, such as internal bleeding and even death.

- *Newsweek* (Dec. 12, 2005) reported, "Nurses are the key to safety in hospitals and nursing homes. You are not admitted to the hospital for medical care but for nursing care."

- ABC World News Tonight (Jan. 21, 2006) reported, "Patients in hospitals today are sicker than 20 years ago."

- The American Hospital Association 2006 Survey reported, "Hospitals face workforce shortages that are affecting patient care. Lawsuit abuse has caused medical liability premiums to rise, disrupting many of the nation's hospitals' ability to provide… services for the communities that depend on them."

Robert Adair, MD, Santa Monica, CA, said, "Medicare and insurance companies don't really cover what care costs. All hospitals are walking a fine line on being insolvent."

Your involvement will help in very specific ways to get your loved one out of the hospital alive. As soon as you apply the information in this book, the patient will be the recipient of your support to ensure their safety and well-being. Keep your eye on one goal: *to support the best possible medical care for your loved one.*

The greatest antidote to a state of helplessness is knowledge. This book will give you the basic knowledge so you can feel familiar with the territory and be more effective in helping your loved one.

Remember:
Your goal is to support the
best possible medical care
for your loved one.

Family's Story

Stewart's wife was in the hospital for colon cancer. He reported that his experience at a major teaching hospital was generally a good one. But he admits that it may have been in part because he was so involved with his wife's care.

Nurses missed a number of things. For example, they'd told me that they wanted to get her up and walking. I asked the next day and no one had helped her out of bed. I did that myself. There were other issues, such as no one taking overall charge. No one was seeing if they were performing the functions. No one was manning the ship. Maybe they were responding to patients making the most noise. So I decided to stay on top of things. I talked to the nurses repeatedly. On the surgical floor, everyone minimized the fact that Danielle wasn't eating. Her strength deteriorated. I decided to take it upon myself to encourage her to eat.

Stewart also said, "I relied on the nurses for the most part. I asked, I pushed, I got second opinions from medical relatives. I became Danielle's advocate."

The Quick Reference Guide and Daily Progress Notes sections are created specifically for your notes. Use them. You should record all essential information there for convenient reference.

You may think that you'll remember every detail of your conversations with the patient's doctors and nurses, but I can almost promise you, you won't. Write everything down in this book. By being present and proactive, you will be able to make positive changes in the way care is delivered to your loved one and contribute to their getting out of the hospital alive.

CHAPTER 2

Getting Started:
The Basics of Being an Advocate

If I'm ever a patient in the hospital, I want a family member there 24/7. It's not that the nurses are incompetent, they are just overworked. **KATHY, RN, BUDA, TX**

WHETHER YOU ARE IN THE EMERGENCY ROOM, the ICU, the Cardiac Wing, Pediatrics, or Med Surg, all of the following steps apply.

There is space for short notes at the end of this chapter. Write the most essential information in the Quick Reference Guide at the end of this book. You will need to refer to this information later.

You might feel completely overwhelmed right now, anxious about what is happening to your loved one, and at a loss as to what to do. Take a deep breath and know that you and your loved one will get through this. You are not alone. Even though you may not know the doctors and nurses who are treating your loved one, they do care and want to do the best job they can. Your input will help them do that.

Perry A. Henderson, MD, Professor Emeritus, Department of Obstetrics and Gynecology, University of Wisconsin Medical School, Madison, WI, said, "Don't allow your loved one to go into the hospital and just let things happen to him."

Your involvement will help your loved one's recovery. Most doctors and nurses I interviewed said, "Patients recover faster when family is involved."

STEP 1

Contact Your Loved One's Family Physician

If your loved one was admitted to the emergency room by someone other than their primary physician, contact the primary physician immediately. If he or she is not on call, your loved one may be seen by a colleague in the practice.

If your loved one's primary doctor does not have privileges at the hospital, you and your loved one have a choice. When you speak to the physician on the phone, ask if the patient should be transferred to a hospital he or she is associated with. Take notes on all of the conversations with the doctor.

"Going to a medical school affiliated hospital is recommended," said Howard S. Traisman, MD, Emeritus Professor of Pediatrics, Northwestern University, Feinberg School of Medicine and Emeritus Attending Endocrinologist, Children's Memorial Hospital, Chicago, IL.

A medical school affiliated hospital isn't necessary, but is recommended by several physicians.

STEP 2

Once the Patient Is Settled, Record Physicians' Information

If the patient is to remain where they are, write the primary care physician's name and phone number in the Quick Reference Guide at the back of this book, page 150. This doctor is in charge of your loved one's case and will be your main contact. Ask how they want to be contacted, and if they will be speaking with any other doctors involved in the case.

If you are in a general hospital, your loved one may be seen by a hospitalist (doctor in charge of patients for the hospital) or an intensivist (doctor in charge of patients in the ICU). If you are in a teaching hospital, your loved one may be seen by the attending, a fellow, a resident, or an intern. Or all of the above. Write down the names, phone numbers, and titles of each doctor. You will refer to this later, especially if more than one doctor is involved.

Ask which doctor is in charge and how to reach him or her.

STEP 3

Assign One Point Person

As the primary advocate for your loved one, you will be the point person, responsible for communicating with doctors and nurses. Every interviewed doctor and nurse emphasized the importance of having one point person. Because nurses and doctors are inundated with patients and paperwork,

Each family/patient should inform the MD of who they have designated to represent them. If the doctor has to discuss treatment decisions with everyone in the family whenever they happen to show up, the MD will not be pleased. The nightmare family is one where everyone wants to share their experiences and opinions about medical care with the doctor.

KAREN BLANCHARD, MD,
SANTA MONICA, CA

they cannot field calls from various family members or friends without taking time away from caring for their patients.

Information about patient diagnosis, prognosis, and progress also becomes watered down and misconstrued when more than one person is involved in the communication.

As your loved one's advocate, you will be the person to communicate with the doctors and nurses and disseminate that information to family members and friends. Write your name and contact information in the Quick Reference Guide, page 144. You can enlist another family member or friend to create a regular email report that is sent to those who are concerned. This cuts down on phone calls to you. Your goal is to reduce as much outside interference as possible. Learn to delegate.

If you are too upset and anxious to delegate, ask a friend or family member to help you do this. You'd be surprised how willing people are to help.

If you are extremely upset by your loved one's medical crisis, consider asking an additional family member to sit in on meetings with doctors and nurses to help sift through the information conveyed. Ask them to write notes in this book about the conversations.

STEP 4

Create a Family Advocate Team

If you cannot be as available as you'd like to act as your loved one's sole advocate, create a Family Advocate Team. Ask if one or two family members or close friends have the time to come by the hospital once or twice a day. Schedule shifts so that each member has an appointed time to visit the patient. Each member of the Family Advocate Team will serve as the patient's eyes and ears. You will be sharing this job with them. There is space in the Quick Reference Guide, page 151, for you to keep track of team members' names and contact information.

Keep in mind, however, that HIPAA privacy laws will affect how much information can be divulged to members of the team (see Chapter 15 for details on patient privacy laws). The patient can request that the Family Advocate Team members' names be placed in the chart so doctors and nurses will know to speak to them.

Leave a copy of this book for team members in the patient's room and ask each to read it. Ask them to take notes on the patient's health status and on any conversations with the primary nurse or doctor. These notes should be written in the Daily Progress Notes pages at the back of this book. Ask them to put their initials next to their notes. Ask members to monitor medications and dosages, and to take notes on any abnormalities with lab work, tests, and procedure results. Each team member will check and update this progress report every day.

With the use of email and phone calls, it should be fairly simple to keep in daily contact with your other support advocates.

Ask friends and family members not to call the hospital or the doctors.

If you do not have family members or friends who can act as support advocates, you might consider hiring a private duty nurse, a sitter, or companion.

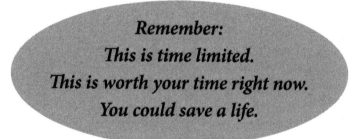

Remember:
This is time limited.
This is worth your time right now.
You could save a life.

STEP 5

Record Current and New Medications

Your loved one's primary physician may be able to give you a computer printout of the patient's medications and medical problems. If that is an option, it will make your job easier.

If it's after hours or a printout isn't available, create a list of medications that your loved one is currently taking. Record this information in the Quick Reference Guide, page 145. Make sure you have the name of the medication and the dosage strength and what condition it is for. The shape and color of the pill doesn't tell the nurse enough.

If you don't have the information, call someone who can get it for you immediately. If your loved one's pharmacy is open, call it. If it's during business hours, call your loved one's family physician's office and ask the nurse there to look up current medications in the patient's chart. Call a family member or friend to bring your loved one's medication bottles from home. Give a copy of this list to the patient's primary nurse and ask that it be placed in the chart.

Be sure to include over-the-counter medications, herbs, and vitamins. They can interact with medications.

You will become familiar with all the medications your loved one is now taking. What shape and color are the pills? What IV medication is the patient on? What is it for? If something changes, ask why. Any change in treatment is probably ordered by the doctor, but mistakes do happen. You want to be aware of any potential mistakes as they occur. Not after.

Several doctors and nurses suggested researching the side effects of any new medications the patient is on. Often, sedation can be a side effect of medication. Is your loved one more listless? It may be due to a new medication or a drug interaction. Ask questions.

STEP 6

Record Known Allergies

Make a list of any known allergies to medications that the patient has experienced. Write them down in the Quick Reference Guide, page 145, and make sure the information is in the patient's chart.

STEP 7

List Current Symptoms, Past Illnesses, and Surgeries

Make a list of current symptoms and problems for your loved one, including recent procedures, illnesses, and any hospital admissions. Record this in the Quick Reference Guide. List which doctor they were treated by and what the treatment was. Give all this information to the primary nurse and ask that it be placed in the patient's chart.

If your loved one is elderly, don't write off symptoms to old age. Inform the primary nurse and primary care doctor of any mood changes, memory loss, change in eating patterns, or speech problems.

STEP 8

Record and Monitor Baseline Vital Signs and Document Lab Tests and Procedures

Become familiar with the patient's vital signs (temperature, pulse, respiration, blood pressure). Record baseline information in the Quick Reference Guide, page 146. If you don't know what the normal ranges for these signs are, ask. If your loved one has high blood pressure, keep your eye on that. Hospital personnel monitor patient vital signs on an on-going basis. You need not record every one of these, but do monitor the vital signs, and note any abnormalities or changes in the Daily Progress Notes.

Depending on the nature of your loved one's illness or injury, various lab tests, x-rays, and procedures may be ordered by the primary doctor and/or attending specialists. If you don't understand why the test or procedure is planned or what it is for, ask.

You may or may not be granted access to the patient's chart. If not, ask the primary nurse questions and write down the answers in this book. Becoming familiar with what is normal for the patient is what counts. Keep your eye on anything that deviates from that norm.

STEP 9

Record the Treatment Plan

Become very familiar with the treatment plan for your loved one. Describe it on the page provided in the Quick Reference Guide. Listen to the doctor and the primary nurse and write down the exact course they plan to take.

Carter Dillman, MD, New York, NY, strongly emphasized this: "When the health plan deviates from the planned course, get involved and ask questions."

STEP 10

Record the Patient's Diet

Monitoring the patient's meals is an important part of being an effective advocate for your loved one. If they are supposed to have a soft diet, watch for meals that aren't soft. If you have a Family Advocate Team, all of you should be on the lookout for dietary mistakes— inadvertent mistakes of course. The hospital is hectic, the kitchen is extremely busy, and it's easy to mix up patients' dietary needs.

Ask the primary nurse what kind of diet the patient is supposed to be on. Record it in the Quick Reference Guide. Check every day and ask your loved one about the meals that have been delivered.

Also watch for the patient's intake of meals. If your loved one isn't feeling well, they may need encouragement to eat. Nurses may be too busy to be on top of this at all times. This is where you can help.

However, Dr. David Wellisch, Chief Psychologist, Adult Division, David Geffen School of Medicine, UCLA, Los Angeles, CA, said, "Do not nudge the patient to eat endlessly. That is the way some families feel effective. But the patient can get overwhelmed by this."

If your loved one is diabetic, check the meal tray for a diabetic meal. If they are given desserts, bring this up to the primary nurse. If a diabetic patient needs to eat several times a day, oversee that snacks are delivered on a regular basis. Ask the patient's primary nurse if you can bring in meals and snacks from home.

STEP 11

Pay Attention — You Are Your Loved One's Eyes and Ears

You will become familiar with your loved one's general health status day by day. If you are paying attention, you will notice if something is different or if your loved one doesn't seem to be doing well. Be proactive. Ask questions. Tune in to what is out of the ordinary. Over 250,000 deaths in the U.S. are blamed on preventable hospital errors. Record your observations in the Daily Progress Notes section. If you find an error has occurred in your loved one's treatment or if you suspect problems, note these in the Errors and Problems section in the Quick Reference Guide.

As your loved one's personal advocate, you are their eyes and ears during their hospitalization. You may think this is not as important

Nurse's Story

Maria, a nurse who works in a teaching hospital, told me this story:

My patient was seen by the intern that morning. The intern wrote in the chart that he was to be discharged that day. That didn't sound right to me. I called the attending. The attending said he was scheduled to have surgery.

Not every nurse can catch these errors. Several nurses mentioned that sometimes the right hand doesn't know what the left hand is doing if there is more than one doctor involved. So why not support the medical care of your loved one and ask questions? If a doctor decides that surgery, a procedure or treatment, or even discharge is necessary, ask questions. When you show up during doctors' rounds you can ask, "Why is this necessary? Why now? I thought that Dr. So-and-So said yesterday that (patient name) needed such and such."

You can ask these questions in very respectful ways without being belligerent. You can soft-pedal the question by saying, "I'm not trying to doubt you, but I just want to be sure. Bear with me..."

in the ICU or Neonatology because of the high nurse-to-patient ratio and the higher training of the nurses on staff there, but many doctors and nurses I spoke to reported that these units are the most important places for a family member to be involved because of the severity of the medical conditions.

Many nurses said that a family member often knows the patient better than the nurses and doctors do. If you see that your loved one isn't doing well, ask questions and talk to the primary nurse. For example: "Mary seemed better yesterday. Today she seems listless." You may discover that there is a new primary nurse on board who wasn't aware that Mary wasn't listless yesterday.

This is how monitoring medical care begins. By checking what is unusual, out of the ordinary or unexpected, you are more apt to catch errors.

STEP 12

Insist on Pain Management

Several physicians suggested that family members insist on pain management for the patient. If your loved one is in pain, speak to the primary care physician about it and ask them to order pain medication. Make sure that the order makes its way into the patient's chart. That way, the nurse won't have to call the physician to get an OK every time the patient is in pain.

STEP 13

Take Special Care if the Patient Is Bedridden

If the patient is unable to get out of bed, ask the primary nurse if he or she has been turned and how often. Bedsores are a common problem for immobile patients. The nurse may have gotten busy with another patient's crisis and may have overlooked it. Make sure you are paying attention.

> ### *Nurse's Story*
>
> Marilyn, an RN from Chicago, told me this story:
>
> *My daughter, Nancy, had eye surgery at age 5. A renal specialist came in and said, 'I'm here to see Nancy.' I asked if there was something wrong with my daughter's kidneys. It turned out there was another Nancy, with a very similar last name, in a hospital room down the hall.*

STEP 14

Catch Patient Name Errors

To prevent patient name errors, ask questions. Any time you encounter a new physician, nurse, or technician, check the patient's name with the medical professional before interaction with the patient begins. For example, if a technician comes to pick up your loved one for a procedure, ask for the name of the patient he or she is coming for and for what procedure. You will have written down the information in this book so you can always reference it.

STEP 15

Speak Up

Every RN I interviewed said that patients and their loved ones are often intimidated by the doctors and nurses. If you are confused about something, ask questions. You have a right to ask questions and feel comfortable with the medical care provided. Make sure your loved one is comfortable as well. If the patient is confused, talk to the primary nurse (no other nurse will do) or doctor and make sure your questions are answered.

Since hospitals can be frantic places because of the number of patient emergencies, it is possible your loved one could be forgotten or overlooked. If your loved one was supposed to receive pain medication

Family's Story

Gail's mother was admitted to a hospital in New York. Here is what she said:

> There were horrible, life-threatening holes with regard to hospital processes and procedures—mistakes with medication, delays with procedures and treatments, hospital politics regarding who got to decide which patients were treated first. There was lack of "team" communication between physicians, nurses, and administrators. Also delayed or no response to nurse call buttons, lack of attention to my mother's skin/body condition. We finally hired a private duty aide to care for her at night when we were not there.
>
> It is frightening to think about those patients who were not lucky enough to have family at their sides. The head nurse was particularly helpful, more so because she saw how dedicated we were. It was sad to hear that our behavior was so unusual.

These situations occur all the time. Even at the best hospitals. Pay attention, because your loved one cannot.

and hasn't, find the primary nurse on the floor and ask questions. If your loved one was supposed to have a procedure and hasn't, ask questions. Don't be surprised, however, if a procedure or surgery has been delayed.

Speaking up in a firm but respectful manner will get you more of what you want for the patient. Even if an error has been made, acting in a belligerent manner will backfire for both you and the patient.

Remember:
Your goal is to support the best possible medical care for your loved one.

If a nurse is administering medications, treatments, injections, or IV solutions to your loved one, ask questions.

Sample questions

1. What is that for?

2. What medication is that?

3. Would you please recheck the name of that medication?

4. Do you know that (name of patient) has an allergic reaction to (name of medication)?

5. (Patient) has (name of illness, injury, or problem). I just wanted to make sure you were aware. I know how busy it can get in the ER.

6. My loved one is in pain. Do you think you could get some medication as soon as possible?

Pain management is extremely important. Make it part of your job to monitor this and contact the primary nurse, repeatedly if necessary, to get your loved one pain medication.

When decisions have been made about your loved one's diagnosis, treatment, or surgical procedures, take notes in this book about what each doctor and primary nurse has said.

We all tend to put blind faith in the hospital, doctors, and nurses and brush aside our instincts. Trust yours. You may know the patient better than any medical professional in the hospital does. Speak up.

STEP 16

Communicate with Staff
About Language and Cultural Issues

If your loved one doesn't speak English, you can help by translating for them. Doctors and nurses cannot do their job if they cannot communicate

Nurse's Story

Jackie, a registered nurse from Stanton, CA, told me a story about a man who was a patient in the ICU. His culture did not allow his face to be touched by a woman. Jackie said,

> Until the patient's wife informed me of this, I tried several times to clean his face, but he became extremely agitated. Nurses in general are educated on cultural preferences and biases but not every nurse knows every detail. It is your job to inform them.

with you or your loved one. Hospitals all have an interpreter who speaks several languages, but often just one for the entire hospital. There are also translation services available by phone. Every patient is legally entitled to translation services. However, if time is of the essence, you can assist. It is in your loved one's best interest to do so.

If your loved one will not eat certain hospital foods for cultural reasons, inform the primary nurse. Make sure the information gets into the patient's chart. Monitor the food yourself. If there has been a mistake, simply bring it to the primary nurse's attention. Be respectful. There may have been a mistake in the kitchen or there may be a new nurse on shift who just didn't know.

Chapter 9 provides additional information on language barriers and cultural issues. A page for your notes on cultural preferences and issues is provided in the Quick Reference Guide.

Notes

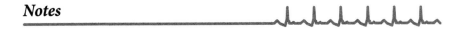

Notes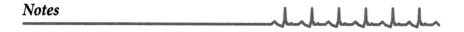

CHAPTER 3

The Primary Nurse

One of the things I love about being a nurse is that I get to care for patients in so many ways. There's nothing like interfacing with patients in their most vulnerable moments. You can't be in nursing and not have an appreciation for those moments.　　　**AMY, RN, OAKLAND, CA**

WHETHER YOUR LOVED ONE IS IN THE ICU, the Step-Down Unit, Cardiac Wing, Med Surg, Pediatrics, etc., one of your first contacts will be the primary nurse. He or she is your loved one's lifeline as well as your own. The primary nurse is the only person who is responsible for the daily care of your loved one and who knows what is going on. You and the patient may see the primary physician infrequently, but the primary nurse is always there to address concerns, answer questions, and respond to the patient's needs.

Many techs, orderlies, and nurses dress alike. Check their name tags. There is going to be a different nurse during the day shift and on the night shift, and there can be a different primary nurse every single day. Be sure to record each primary nurse's name, direct phone number, and other relevant information in the Physician/Nurse/Specialist section of the Quick Reference Guide. Remember: Only ask questions of the patient's primary nurse or doctor, no one else.

The primary nurses' names and those of other nurses involved in your loved one's case may be written on a board in the patient's room. Check the board when you arrive each day so that you know who is responsible for care on the current shift.

If a medical professional comes into the patient's room and you don't see a nametag, ask for their name. Ask what they do in the hospital.

Be nice and polite.

STEP 1

Introduce Yourself to the Primary Nurse

Introduce yourself to the primary nurse as the patient's family member and point person. Express that you will be conducting all communication for the patient's family and friends and relaying information to them. Be charming and respectful of the primary nurse.

Even if they haven't responded to the patient's call button in a timely manner or have seemed abrupt or have made you wait, maintain your likeable personality. Many interviewed nurses revealed that too often a belligerent or disrespectful family member causes nurses to avoid them. This translates to less attention to the patient.

Remember:
Your goal is to support the
best possible medical care
for your loved one.

Nurse's Story

Yolanda, a registered nurse from the Midwest, shared a story about a patient's family member who had asked an orderly for pain medication for her mother. Apparently the family member didn't realize that the primary nurse was responsible for giving medications or didn't know who the patient's primary nurse was. The family member finally approached the primary nurse and was extremely upset. She explained that she'd asked for medication for her mother forty-five minutes earlier, and her mother was in terrible pain. Yolanda explained to me that family members are frequently confused about this.

Know who your loved one's primary nurse is. Only ask this person for pain medication.

STEP 2

Establish a Relationship

Ask the primary nurse to explain the patient's diagnosis, plan of treatment, and all medications that are currently being administered. Write down all responses in the back of this book.

At the end of the initial conversation, it is in your best interest as well as that of your loved one, to ask the nurse if there is anything you can do to help. They may give you a list or simply tell you to be there as much as possible. By asking questions and initiating discussions, you are establishing a very important relationship with the nurse. You want him or her to see you as an involved family member.

Offer appreciation for what the nurses are doing. There may be a different primary nurse on each shift every day. If this is the case, go through the routine of introducing yourself, asking what you can do to help, and showing thanks to each and every one. This will pay off for your loved one.

STEP 3

Divulge All Patient Information

Most interviewed registered nurses mentioned the importance of family members divulging all pertinent information about the patient to the primary nurse. Sometimes, patients don't want to reveal bad habits, without realizing that these habits could affect medications, procedures, tests, or treatments. Or the patient may have simply forgotten something. If you are having a conversation with the primary nurse and you realize that the patient has omitted something, bring it up, either in the room with the patient or after you leave the room. All information about the patient is vital to their care.

STEP 4

Respect Your Loved One's Privacy

You might also consider stepping out of the room to give the patient privacy if they want to speak to the nurse alone. Some patients want to save face and will not divulge all information if you are present.

STEP 5

How to Interact with the Primary Nurse

Nurses are saints. Most love their work. They are the primary caregivers on a daily basis for your loved one. Treat them with respect and kindness. If not out of humanity alone, then do it for your loved one. If you want more attention for your loved one, be kind and show appreciation to the primary nurse. The more courteous you are, the more likely it is that your loved one will receive needed attention.

One interviewed nurse said this: "Sometimes family members are unreasonable and expect perfection. I just wish for a little more understanding from them when the floor is understaffed."

Only speak to your loved one's primary nurse about any patient needs. If the patient needs pain medication, is in distress, or needs immediate attention, call the primary nurse or find them on the floor. Be courteous and tell them what is wrong.

Many RNs, LVNs, CNAs, lab techs, and other medical staff dress alike. Since you have written down the name of your loved one's primary nurse, it will be easier for you to track them down. Do not ask any other nurse or medical professional (other than the patient's doctor) for answers to questions, pain medication, or help with patient distress. To prevent unnecessary confusion, know whom to speak to: the patient's primary nurse or doctor. No one else.

> *I love being a nurse. I've never worked harder in my life. Helping patients is the best aspect of the job. Finishing my day, knowing I've made a difference, keeps me going.* KATHY, RN, BUDA, TX

STEP 6

Know When the Primary Nurses Change Shift

There are two times a day when primary nurses report to the new primary nurses who are coming on duty. This is when they go over each patient's chart and health status. This is the only time they have to share information about the patients and to bring the new primary nurses up to speed. Find out when nurse shift change is, and do not bother them then if possible. Most nurses said that it is best not to be on the floor when nurse shift change occurs.

Several interviewed nurses and social workers had this to say: "If nurses are setting limits around their availability during shift change, it's not personal. It's about the care of the patient. They are putting the patient first."

STEP 7

Get Involved

The primary nurse is there to fully care for your loved one. It would behoove you to ask the nurse how you can help care for the patient. List what you can do, such as helping the patient to the bathroom, bringing them ice chips or water, propping them up in bed, walking them down the hall if appropriate, changing bedding, or assisting with a bath. Ask if you can place a cold washcloth on your loved one's head.

Ask what you can bring into the hospital room from home, such as photos, MP3 player, CD player, pajamas, or personal hygiene items (see Chapter 12, "How to Support and Comfort Your Loved One").

Asking the primary nurse what you can do to help not only benefits your loved one, but it will also show the nurse a very important aspect of yourself that will establish your relationship and benefit the patient: that you want to be involved.

Almost every nurse I interviewed said that patients with loved ones who are involved get more attention. It's human nature.

STEP 8

Humanize the Patient

Some nurses said that the patient becomes more of a real human being to them when they see family members helping out. Tell the nurse about your loved one. The more the nurse can see your loved one as a person with a story, with a history, with a family and friends, the more attention your loved one will get. Nurses see patients all day long, week after week, and it is normal for them to become somewhat immune to the suffering they see. They have to, in order to cope with their job.

You want the primary nurse to see your loved one not as one of the thousands of patients that come through the unit each year, but as a human being.

A personal connection with the primary nurse is what you want for your loved one. If you have to initiate that because your loved one is too ill, then do everything you can to tell the nurse about him. What he does for a living, what his interests are, whether he has children or grandchildren. Try to find some common ground. If the primary nurse loves dogs, tell him or her about your loved one's dog and how much he loves it.

A personal connection can promote better care.

Almost all of the RNs said, "Tell me something about the patient. It helps me see them as a human being with a family, with a job, with children, with interests. I just get so overwhelmed sometimes that it's all I can do to keep up with caring for my patients. If I know something about them, it helps me to connect with them."

One registered nurse, Jackie, said, "The more we know about the patients, the better care we can render."

STEP 9

Bring Cookies and Candy

If your loved one has been in the hospital even for only a couple of days, consider bringing in cookies, candy, or healthy snacks for the nurses. Be sure to put a thank you card with your name and your loved one's name on it and attach it to the box or basket. This basket or box will be placed on the nursing station counter. No one will know who it is from unless you permanently attach an open-face gift card with your name and the patient's name. Thank them for all they are doing to care for your loved one.

STEP 10

Understand that Nurses Must Spend Time Charting

Many nurses explained that family members get upset when they see them seated at the nurses' station. Often nurses are doing what is called "charting." The hospital requires that nurses document everything that happens to a patient—each medication given, each blood pressure reading, each meal eaten—as well as their observations about how each patient is doing. It takes up a lot of time. So, before you lose your temper because you see a nurse seated at the nurses' station, check to see if they are charting.

STEP 11

How to Handle a Problem With the Nurse

If there is a problem with any nurse who is involved in your loved one's care, each and every nurse I interviewed said to speak to the primary nurse first. Do not go over their head without initially speaking to them. Talk to them calmly about what the problem is and how you hope it can be solved. Be respectful and firm, not belligerent.

Don't be frightened to speak up because you are afraid it will negatively affect the patient. This is your job. You would do it for your child. Do it for your loved one.

If you have noticed a repeated problem with a primary nurse and how they care for your loved one, ask the nurse supervisor (the nurse who supervises the activities of the nursing department), the nurse manager (the nurse who handles all the problems on the unit), or the charge nurse (the person responsible for supervising all primary nurses and can help solve problems for families and patients) to make a change. The hospital may also have a patient advocate who can help you. Tell this person you would like a different primary nurse to care for your loved one. Remember to be firm but respectful. Explain the problem. Define how you would like it to be resolved. Do not threaten. This will backfire. Ask the nurse supervisor or charge nurse to put a notation of your request in the patient's chart.

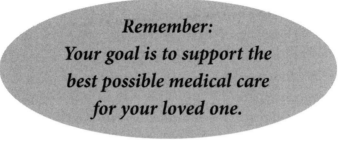

Remember:
Your goal is to support the
best possible medical care
for your loved one.

STEP 12

Consider Hiring a Private Duty Nurse, Caregiver, Companion, or Sitter

Karen Blanchard, MD, offered this observation: "Nighttime is an especially vulnerable time for many elderly patients, and they should be asked if they want someone to stay overnight. This might require a private room."

Most nurses suggested hiring private duty nurses for every patient at night, on holidays, and on weekends. Many even suggested having them 24/7, regardless of the time of day or day of the week.

Having a private duty nurse, if you can afford it, is especially beneficial at night, when the ratio of nurses to patients goes down, meaning that there are fewer nurses to care for your loved one.

Most interviewed doctors and nurses suggested hiring a sitter, a private duty nurse, or a companion if the patient is confused, very ill, or if it's a holiday, weekend, or summer month.

Perry A. Henderson, MD, Professor Emeritus, University of Wisconsin Medical School, Madison, WI, suggested hiring one of these professionals if the patient is in a rural hospital because the ratio of nurses to patients is frequently lower there.

Keep in mind that in some states, private duty nurses may not legally be able to do any more than a family member can. In this case, hiring a sitter, caregiver, or companion would be the best option. The hospital will let you know if it even allows private duty nurses in the hospital. Ask questions.

If you decide to hire someone, ask the hospital for referrals. It is particularly helpful if your loved one has a private nurse, companion, or sitter who is already connected to the hospital and familiar with the hospital's routine. If they don't give you referrals, you can find a sitter through a domestic agency. This person will be there to watch out for your loved one and help with things such as getting him or her to the bathroom, alerting the primary nurse if the patient is in need, or helping them sip water, etc.

Following are general fees (these may change at any time).

- **Private Duty Nurses (RNs):** $55-65 per hour and time-and-a-half for holidays.

- **LVNs:** $44 per hour with time-and-a-half for holidays.

- **Nurse's Aides:** $22-30 per hour with time-and-a-half for holidays.

- **Caregivers:** $20-21 per hour.

Most insurance companies do not cover the cost of private duty nurses.

One family member, Emily, hired a sitter after her husband tried to pull out his IV so that he could get up and go to the bathroom. He had pressed the buzzer for the nurse and no one had arrived. After several tries, he gave up. "Someone needs to be there," Emily said. "Do not rely on the hospital for full care."

Robert Adair, MD, Santa Monica, CA, said this: "If the hospital looks like it's not staffed appropriately or if a patient is confused, a sitter or private duty nurse is very helpful. A family member being there with the patient is better than nothing."

Most family members I interviewed hired sitters for loved ones at night. Almost everyone recommended hiring a sitter if a patient is confused.

Family's Story

Nadia lived in Southern California. Her father lived in Phoenix, where he was hospitalized. She traveled to see him once a week in the hospital. She noticed that the nurses were taking care of too many patients and she worried about what happened when she traveled back to her home to be with her children. Nadia didn't know that she could have hired a sitter or nurse for evenings and weekends to oversee his care. Her father passed away from pneumonia while she was home. She said she will never know if she could have helped to prevent the progression of that disease if she'd hired someone to be there with him when she could not.

STEP 13

Consider Sharing a Private Duty Nurse with Another Family

A pediatrician, Lucy Hu Bruttomesso, MD, suggested, "Two families in a semi-private room may be able to get together and hire a private duty nurse and share the cost. But check with the hospital first to find out if this is permissible."

STEP 14

What to Do if You Can't Afford a Private Duty Nurse or Sitter

If you cannot afford a full-time private duty nurse or sitter, you might consider hiring one just for a few nights, or on the weekend, or on a holiday. If that is still not an option, consider asking a member of your Family Advocate Team to stay with your loved one.

If that isn't possible, ask a friend, or hire a friend's babysitter or housekeeper and give them this book.

Go over the patient's daily progress notes with them, and tell them everything you want done. Ask them to read relevant chapters of this book.

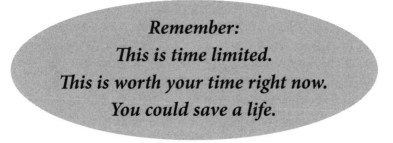

Remember:
This is time limited.
This is worth your time right now.
You could save a life.

STEP 15

Be Aware of the Hospital Nursing Shortage

If a hospital is short on nurses, it will hire temporary nurses from its registries or from outside agencies. If this happens, you and every member of your Family Advocate Team need to be more watchful. These nurses, as honest and motivated as the rest, may not be familiar with the routine at your hospital, and the chance of error may increase.

If your primary nurse is a "traveler," meaning they are hired by a hospital for several weeks at a time, or they are from a registry (a nursing agency or private business that provides per diem nurses to hospitals, medical offices, and individuals), go over all information about your loved one with that nurse. Watch closely. These nurses may have just started their jobs and may not be familiar with a particular hospital's routine.

My last night, I had six patients. I said I had an unsafe patient assignment. I told them I accepted it under protest.

ANONYMOUS RN, PASADENA, CA

Notes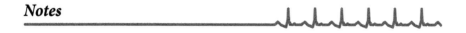

Notes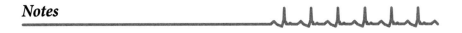

CHAPTER 4

The Doctors

As much as we'd like to be, physicians can't be at the hospital at all times. Someone, a family member, must be at bedside to watch, support, and care.

**ANONYMOUS MD, SAINT JOHN'S MEDICAL CENTER,
SANTA MONICA, CA**

STEP 1

How to Reach the Doctors

If you take one thing from this book, take this: Show up during doctors' rounds for your initial conversation with all the doctors. Wait in your loved one's hospital room until they arrive. Ask the patient's primary nurse when the doctors are to be expected. Plan to sit and wait, especially for your initial visit. You'll want to discuss issues and ask questions in person.

Meeting face-to-face does more than just support clear and effective communication. It also shows the doctors that someone is looking out for your loved one. Every doctor and nurse I interviewed told me that if a family member is involved and shows up on a regular basis, the patient will receive more attention.

Showing up during a doctor's rounds also avoids telephone tag between you and the doctor. That is a source of frustration to many family members and physicians and can so easily be avoided.

First, find out from the primary nurse who the primary care physician is for the patient. Write down their name and phone number in the Physicians/Nurses/Specialists information section of the Quick Reference Guide. This doctor will be the main physician who will be coordinating care if there are other doctors involved, and he will be your main contact.

If you have already had an opportunity to speak with your loved one's primary nurse, then you are one step ahead. You will know a little more and will be able to ask more informed questions of the doctor.

Show up before the appointed time and expect to wait. Doctors are juggling other patients' medical needs and have to respond to emergencies, which cause delays. While you are waiting, create a list of questions with your loved one (if they are cognizant) for the doctors and write them down in the Daily Progress Notes section.

STEP 2

Be Patient While the Doctor Reviews the Chart

If the doctor has just arrived on the floor, give them a chance to read the patient's chart, evaluate the case, and speak to the primary nurse. They can't talk to you until they have. Understandably, you and your loved one are anxious to meet with the doctor. But doctors have to get up to speed with the patient's health status before they can answer any questions.

If you are at a teaching hospital, your loved one will be assigned an attending doctor (the doctor who leads the health-care team). The patient might also be seen by a fellow, a resident, and an intern. It is crucial to meet with all of these physicians in person.

If you are in a general hospital, plan to meet with the intensivist (hospital doctor assigned to take care of all critical care patients in the hospital), or hospitalist (hospital doctor who cares for all hospital patients), or your loved one's primary physician. This is especially important in the beginning. Use the time while you are waiting to create your list of questions with your loved one (if they are able). Write everything down in the Daily Progress Notes section.

STEP 3

How to Have an Effective First Meeting

When the doctor arrives in your loved one's room, introduce yourself. It's common sense that if someone feels comfortable with you, they will be more willing to pay attention and communicate with you. We all have the tendency to get defensive and tense when we are frightened and stressed. Remind yourself that the more respectful you are to the doctor, the more likely it is that they will engage with you and your loved one. You want this person's time and attention in the few minutes they are in your loved one's room. Several interviewed doctors expressed concern over family members acting in a condescending manner.

> *You are not the expert. If you put the doctor on the defensive, you're done. They are afraid of getting sued.*
>
> ANONYMOUS MD, PORTLAND, ME

Ask the doctor how they prefer to be contacted with questions or concerns. This is a key question because it opens the door to reaching them in a more efficient manner. They may give you an office number or cell phone number, or tell you that the primary nurse knows how to reach them. Write down the doctor's phone numbers in the Quick Reference Guide, page 150. Ask if they can be contacted by email. Ask for their business card.

STEP 4

Ask Questions

Every doctor and nurse I spoke with said that involving the patient in their own care is crucial to their well-being. The patient doesn't want to feel helpless and out of control. Being a patient in the hospital is stressful enough.

If you aren't familiar with the medical jargon the physician is using, ask them to use layman's terms. Many family members expressed frustration with doctors using complicated language they did not understand.

Ask the physician to clarify each and every thing you do not understand. Speak up.

Sample questions:

1. What is wrong with my loved one? What is the diagnosis?

2. What is your plan of treatment?

3. What medications are being administered, and what procedures and tests are planned and why?

4. Are the medications the patient is being given now the same as what they have been taking at home? If not, why? (The hospital formulary may not offer the same medication.)

5. Which other doctors (specialists) are involved in my loved one's case? What are their names? When can I expect to meet them? How can I reach them?

6. Who is coordinating care? Who is in charge of my loved one's care?

7. What is the prognosis? How long do you anticipate the patient will be in the hospital?

8. How can I best reach you? How do you prefer I contact you if I have questions or concerns?

Write down the answers to these questions in the Daily Progress Notes section.

If the answer to any of these questions is, "I'm not sure at this point," make a note to follow up with the same question or questions in the next phone call or meeting.

One interviewed family member, Chuck, said, "You have to pin down doctors; find a doctor outside the hospital who will give you a list of questions to ask."

STEP 5

Interact Effectively with the Doctors

Keep in mind that you are going to be proactive, but at the same time, respectful to the doctors. They know what they are doing.

Family members frequently get frustrated when they're unable to reach doctors or don't know which questions to ask, how to communicate with them, or how to establish a relationship that can lead to more attention for the patient.

To interact effectively and efficiently with a physician, do your homework. Have your list of questions prepared ahead of time. It's a good idea to have done a little research so you can discuss the patient's diagnosis and treatment, instead of blindly relying on the physician's expertise. This is not to supersede the doctor's expertise—this is for you—so you can feel more in control and understand what is going on. You want to save time and make the most of the visit. So come prepared.

STEP 6

What to Do if More Than One Doctor Is Involved

Several family members expressed frustration over there being "no captain of the ship," meaning, they didn't feel that there was one main doctor in charge when several specialists were involved in their loved one's case.

Ask the primary care doctor which doctor is coordinating the patient's care. This would be the physician in charge of the patient's case, the one who will be coordinating all the other specialists.

Write down the doctor's name and phone number. Record this information in the Quick Reference Guide. Ask if you might contact them every couple of days for an update. Every time you talk or meet with your loved one's doctor, have your questions ready.

During the conversation with the doctor, write down the answers to your questions. If something doesn't make sense, then ask the doctor to clarify. Don't be afraid to ask questions. Be assertive. You will have a few minutes to go over everything with the doctor and you don't want to waste time. Try not to panic if you think of more questions after the meeting is over. List those questions at the end of this chapter and/or in the Daily Progress Notes.

One of the functions of the primary nurse is to translate information given to you by the doctor. If you don't understand something the doctor has said and you didn't have a chance to ask for clarification, write down the question and ask if the primary nurse has time to go over it with you and your loved one.

Nurse's Story

We had a patient who had two doctors and both were assuming that the other was the primary physician, so getting pain medication was really difficult. I think it's a good idea to ask the doctors what their actual role is and how they are going to participate after the procedure, just so everyone's on the same page.   RACHEL, RN, PORTLAND, OR

STEP 7

What to Do if You Cannot Be There During Doctors' Rounds

If you cannot wait for the doctor to show up during rounds, the next best option is to ask the primary nurse to place a note in the patient's chart asking the doctor to call you during rounds. Follow the previous steps, even in a phone call.

If you are concerned that a doctor might not call or that you might miss their call, ask the primary nurse for the approximate expected time of arrival for the doctor. Call the hospital floor at that time. If you don't reach the doctor, leave a message with the primary nurse that you would like to speak to the doctor as soon as possible and ask that your request be put in the patient's chart.

When you speak to the doctor on the phone, be sure to follow the guidelines about asking how a doctor prefers to be reached. That way, you'll have a better chance of actually connecting with them in the future.

Fran, a medical office manager in Los Angeles, CA, recommended this: "Fax a note to the doctor you want to speak with. Explain that you would like to talk with him/her on the phone. Write down your work hours, your office, cell phone and home phone numbers and times you are available."

If the hospital has a social worker, they may be willing to intervene on your behalf. If you are having trouble reaching a doctor, ask the social worker if they would be willing to call or page the doctor.

STEP 8

How to Handle a Communication Breakdown

Communication with doctors can break down easily for a number of reasons. Here are three:

1. It is a holiday or weekend or both.

2. Your loved one's physician is not on call. This is the time to take a deep breath. Understand that you will be helping to facilitate communication with the physician who is coming in place of your loved one's doctor. Your notes will be crucial to your role as patient advocate.

3. When there is more than one physician involved in your loved one's case.

An MD from Johns Hopkins Hospital in Baltimore, who preferred to remain anonymous, said, "It's always a problem if a different doctor is involved who doesn't know the patient. The worst is at night, if the doctor hasn't seen the patient before. It's not a perfect system, because a doctor can't be on call twenty-four hours a day. When a doctor goes off call, they will give a verbal or written report to the new doctor. The main family member should be there to supplement information relayed by the nurse."

If your loved one's physician is part of a medical group, call the office and find out who will be making hospital rounds and when their rotation will be at the hospital. Show up at the hospital at the anticipated hour or call the nurses' station at that time.

You will have to be on your toes to be sure you document the doctors' names, their visits, who they are covering for, and what each has said about your loved one. Write down their diagnoses and any comments in the Quick Reference Guide, page 148. You will use those notes when you speak to the doctors. You will act as an information

> **Family's Story**
>
> One family member, David, said this:
>
> *There were so many doctors involved in my dad's case. The pulmonologist took me aside and showed me the results of my dad's scan. Because I brought in specific questions, she became more involved.*

facilitator and bring each new physician up to speed based on what you know about the patient.

Fran, a medical office manager in Los Angeles suggests, "Fax a note to the primary physician that says, 'We would like a consultation with you after you have spoken to the other consulting physicians (list names) who are involved with (patient name).'"

You can also put the same note in the patient's chart for the primary physician to read the next time they come onto the hospital floor.

Ask each physician to inform you about their conversations with any other physicians involved. Ask that they contact the other doctors, if that hasn't been done already. Make a note about the physician's answers. If any follow-up needs to be done, you will have it documented in the Daily Progress Notes. Then follow up by calling the doctor's office the next day. Leave a detailed message with the nurse or office manager.

One of the most frustrating situations you might deal with is when there are differing opinions from several doctors involved in your loved one's case.

You'll want to keep track of as many conversations with physicians as you can. Write down pertinent comments from each doctor in the Daily Progress Notes. If opinions about diagnosis or treatment differ, try to get the majority opinion from the patient's primary nurses and physicians about what is happening with your loved one. This is where further research and discussions might help you decide.

Family's Story

    Arlyn's husband had cancer and was a patient in a major teaching hospital. She told me, "All the conflicting opinions with all the specialists was the biggest problem. I never knew who was in charge of my husband's case, who was coordinating all of his treatment." Arlyn said she wouldn't agree to anything until all the doctors involved had reached a consensus.

STEP 9

When Information is Confusing, Ask For a Group Meeting

Karen Blanchard, MD, a surgeon in Santa Monica, CA, suggested this: "Group meetings are helpful when families and/or patients feel they are getting confusing information from different sources. The primary care MD has the responsibility to communicate with the family and patient concerning treatment plans and treatment goals."

    Ask your loved one's primary physician to call a group meeting with the primary nurse and all physicians involved in your loved one's case. You can discuss the differing opinions with each doctor. Take notes about what each one said. Review your notes before you talk again with the doctors later.

STEP 10

When to Get a Second Opinion

If at any time your loved one isn't doing as well as expected, you can ask the patient's primary doctor for a second opinion from another physician. Asking for a second opinion should not offend any doctor. It is your right.

    Fran, the medical office manager in Los Angeles, CA, revealed: "Doctors tend to refer their buddies for second opinions. Be sure that any doctors who are called in to consult are experienced and competent."

A few things to consider when bringing in a consultant:

1. Is the physician board-certified in his or her specialty?

2. Is he or she affiliated with a medical school?

With my own mother's hospitalization, I called in a specialist from the major university in a nearby city. This specialist's observation concurred with those of the other physicians, but I can rest now, knowing that I did everything I could.

Sometimes a second set of eyes can yield an idea your loved one's primary doctor hadn't thought of or hadn't yet considered, or it can yield a more honed diagnosis and ideas for further treatments.

Leslie, an RN from Lakewood, CA, said, "Family members can ask nurses for recommendations for medical staff who might perform procedures." She suggested posing the question like this, "Who do you think has the most experience doing this?"

STEP 11

Schedule a Pre-op Visit if Your Loved One Needs an Operation

If an operation is scheduled for your loved one, ask the primary care physician and surgeon to schedule pre-op visits with you and the patient. Have your list of questions ready before you meet with them at the appointed times.

Sample questions:

1. What is the operation, exactly?

2. What is the anticipated outcome?

3. What does recovery look like?

4. Will there be any special dietary needs after the operation?

5. Are there additional medications my loved one will be taking?

6. What are the risks?

7. Does my loved one know about the risks?

8. Would you, yourself, please mark the incision site with a permanent marker?

When a technician comes to pick up your loved one for an operation, ask for the name of the patient they are coming for and the name of the operation the patient is scheduled for.

Go with the patient to the operating room. You will not be able to enter the room itself, but you might see the surgeon and other medical staff. Review with the surgeon and other medical staff what the operation is and the location on the patient's body where the incision will be made.

For example: Your loved one is having a shoulder operation. Check to be sure they have the correct patient's name. Ask that the surgeon himself mark the incision site with a permanent marker on the patient's body. Check to be sure the correct shoulder is marked.

If you interact with anesthesiologists, surgical nurses, and radiologists before the surgery, go over the name of the surgery and the location of the incision site on the patient's body.

Ask where to wait for the surgeon after the operation so they don't have to spend valuable time looking for you.

STEP 12

Optimize the Doctor/Patient/ Family Member Relationship

We are all groomed to view doctors as superhuman experts. Many of us are also taught to believe that we must allow them to do their jobs and not interfere with questions. Because of that one-up-one-down relationship, we all need to keep in mind that yes, they are the experts, and yes, they are fully capable of taking care of our loved one. But we must also remind ourselves that we as family members are contributors to the health and well-being of the patient.

Several doctors and many nurses reported that family members are intimidated by physicians and prefer to ask questions of the primary nurse instead of the physicians. This is a time when you must step out of your comfort zone and be proactive. Here are several common beliefs and reasons to reconsider them:

1. **I don't want to bother the doctor.** Don't wait for the doctors to call you. Be assertive. Wait for them in the patient's room during rounds. Several interviewed nurses said, "Sometimes family members think they have to turn over their loved one to the staff and they don't do anything for the patient themselves. Or they're afraid that if they do, it will interfere with their loved one's medical care." Not so. Support the nursing caregivers, be a sentinel, and provide patient comfort. Ask questions of the doctors and primary nurses. It is your right.

2. **I don't understand what is going on.** If you don't understand something about what is being done with your loved one, ask questions.

3. **I'm intimidated by the doctor.** It is normal to feel a little intimidated by a physician, who has so much more knowledge about a specific area than you do, but this is your loved one we are talking about. Blind faith in a physician will rarely

Remember:
You are the eyes and ears for your loved one. If you take on the job as advocate, your loved one will be much better off for it.

contribute to your loved one's well-being, nor will it facilitate communication about the patient's progress or status. Speak up. You probably know a lot about the patient that can help with their treatment and care.

STEP 13

Schmooze the Physician

Keep in mind that when questioning a doctor, it is all in the presentation. Doctors are too busy to deal with overly demanding family members, and they don't want to. So the important part of setting the stage for a successful relationship with the physician is to be respectful, to listen carefully to what they have to say, take notes, do your research, and schmooze. Yes, schmooze. Be polite, friendly, and establish a mutual foundation of respect. If you complain and are consistently negative, without expressing appreciation for their hard work and any successes with your loved one, you may cause the physician to shut down. It's human nature.

STEP 14

How to Get What You Want

A number of interviewed nurses reported that some family members treat doctors and nurses like indentured servants. This is just not smart. Of course you are upset over the state of your loved one. Maybe there have even been medical errors or delays with pain medication and treatment.

Keep in mind that these medical professionals are offering your loved one premium care and treatment that you, yourself cannot offer. They have something you want.

The effective way to go after what you want is to be assertive, respectful, and polite. Think about salespeople: you are more inclined to buy what they are selling if you like them as people. In the same way, if a physician likes you, they are more apt to respond favorably. Use your people skills when interacting with them. If you can get them on your side, they will be more likely to go the extra mile for your loved one.

What to Do if the Doctor Doesn't Have a Good Bedside Manner

There are always going to be people who are difficult or arrogant. This applies to doctors as well. They can have bad days or weeks. You may encounter a doctor who thinks the family should be invisible and who wants the space simply to do the work. This situation requires some diplomacy on your part. Think about people you've encountered in your job or at your child's school who are just plain difficult to deal with. The tricky part is, you still need something from them. How do you get it? Becoming arrogant yourself just won't work. Your loved one is in need, and he or she needs a particular kind of care that only a hospital can offer. Make the best of the situation by being firm and assertive, but pleasant.

If a doctor doesn't want to be bothered with your questions, back-pedal your question with something like this: "I'm not doubting you, I'm just unclear about… It seemed that Jim was doing so much better before he received such and such medication or treatment. Is there a possibility that it didn't agree with him? I've just never seen him like this."

The doctor may respond with, "This is the nature of Jim's illness."

Gently, ask again, but use a different approach: "I understand that, and I know you are doing everything you can to help Jim recover. I read about Jim's illness (or talked to another physician), and I just wondered if such and such could be happening. I'm sure you've thought of this already. Just thought I'd run it by you."

If you are making no headway with the doctor who has the lousy bedside manner, your next option is to speak to another doctor involved in your loved one's case. This is not an effort to backstab the doctor who has the lousy bedside manner, but to appeal to the other doctor's sympathy. Doctors protect one another, so don't alienate any of them.

Here's a way to go about it: "I have spoken with (name of doctor) and I'm still not clear on what is happening with Jim. Do you have a minute to answer a couple of questions?"

When the doctor says yes, proceed with this: "I was wondering if possibly this medication or treatment could be having a bad effect on Jim. He hasn't seemed the same. Something just doesn't feel right. Do you have any ideas about what might be going on?" Then run your questions by this other doctor. Do not mention that you were dissatisfied in any way with the doctor with the lousy bedside manner. Simply bypass the specifics of your experience and explain that you are confused about something. Ask for the other doctor's input.

> *Remember:*
> *Your goal is to support the*
> *best possible medical care*
> *for your loved one.*

The above guidelines for communicating with doctors may sound like you are being asked to tiptoe around these professionals. This is not the case. You are being urged to ask questions and to be proactive in your loved one's care. But you are also being told about the reality of doctors' work demands and schedules. It is better to be informed so you can work within the confines of their availability rather than to resist what simply cannot be changed.

This thought may still cross your mind: "Wait a minute, this is their job. Treating patients is what they get paid for." These guidelines are to help you circumvent the red tape. Simply get moving and expect to do some of the work yourself.

Notes

Notes

CHAPTER 5

The Importance of Research

Be careful when doing research on the Internet. There's all sorts of scary stuff on it and some information may be inaccurate. **BONNIE, RN, PORTLAND, OR**

THE TIME TO START DOING RESEARCH on your loved one's illness, injury, or surgery is after your initial meeting with the primary nurse. You can do research on the Internet or at a public library, or the hospital may have a library of its own. The hospital may also have a website with information and links. Informative and credible websites are listed in the appendix of this book. You can also ask the primary nurse, doctor, and hospital social worker for a resource list.

Some hospitals will even have information on a hospital channel on the patient's TV.

The importance of research is twofold:

1. Research enables you to have reasonably educated conversations with the doctors and primary nurses about your loved one's illness or injury. You'll be more capable of asking intelligent questions and understanding their answers. This empowers you to be more proactive on behalf of the patient.

    If you have educated yourself, you are much more apt to notice if something goes wrong, such as a medical error.

2. Research lessens some of your own sense of helplessness. There is nothing like a little education and knowledge to make you feel more in control.

STEP 1

Visit the Hospital Library

Ask the primary nurse where the hospital library is. Go there and review the information it offers. You may find pamphlets about your loved one's disease, illness, or injury, or full books and magazines on the subject. The library may also offer support groups and classes.

STEP 2

Visit Internet Websites

Research the websites listed in the appendix of this book. If you have questions after doing research, write them down in the Research section, page 163. If there is a new treatment you've discovered that is being done for the illness or injury that your loved one has, bring it up with the doctor. Your question can sound like this: "I've been doing some research. The Mayo Clinic is doing "x" treatment for the kind of illness/injury Jim has. Do you think that would be appropriate for my husband?"

Be nice and polite.

STEP 3

Seek Out Other Families on the Same Hospital Floor

Many family members reported that their relationship to other families with loved ones on the same hospital floor was invaluable. They were able to exchange researched information and support. Friendships with other family members can be particularly important if you are spending a lot of time in the hospital. Consider reaching out.

Notes

Notes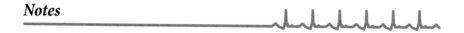

CHAPTER 6

Preventing Medical Error

I would recommend to almost everyone that they try to stay out of hospitals as much as possible. If you need to be in one, have someone with you, around the clock, as your advocate.

ANDREA STEIN, MD, SANTA MONICA, CA

ACCORDING TO THE INSTITUTE OF MEDICINE, "A hospital patient can expect, on average, to be subjected to more than one medication error each day."

Preventing medical errors for your loved one is not a fail-safe task. But there are a number of things you can do to help prevent errors from occurring.

Patients' names get mixed up, surgeons operate on the wrong part of the body, the wrong medications are administered and in the wrong dosages, or a treatment goes wrong. All because people are human. The hospital staff are doing their best. They are not committing medical errors because they want to—that is the last thing they want. But with your involvement, you can help them be more vigilant.

Preventing medical error requires checking and rechecking and asking questions. Don't be afraid to speak up. This issue is publicized in the media, and hospital staff are well aware of how nervous patients and their families are. They welcome your involvement.

STEP 1

Check Medications

Make a list of each pill name and dosage in the Medications section of the Quick Reference Guide, pages 147, 152. Watch for different colors or shapes of pills that are administered to the patient. If a pill looks different or new, ask the primary nurse what the medication is and what it is for. If injections are given, ask the medication name, dosage, and what it is for. Compare the information offered to you with your current records. Ask the nurse to recheck the medication name, as bottles can look alike.

Be polite and ask the nurse respectfully. Tell them you are just trying to make sure there hasn't been an inadvertent mistake. A mistake can also be made by the hospital pharmacy or doctor, not just the nurse.

Check all medications administered to the patient and make sure they have been assigned by the doctor. If you don't understand why a medication has been prescribed, ask questions.

A recent study on a sample of fifty-six hospital intensive care units, done by US Pharmacopoeia, reported that 38,000 medication mistakes occurred in one year.

Sometimes medications have similar names and similar-looking labels and bottles, and mix-ups can easily occur. Doctors' handwriting is notoriously illegible, and it is so easy for a pharmacist to misread the name of the medication. Be sure to check.

Check for any inconsistencies in shape, size, or color of the medications administered to the patient. Ask questions if something looks different.

Patients can also have allergic or adverse reactions to medications. If your loved one starts having any adverse effects after a medication has been given, alert the primary nurse. Stay on top of it. Make notes in the Daily Progress Notes at the back of this book.

Doctor's Story

After having neck surgery, Andrea Stein, MD, Santa Monica, CA, was a patient in a hospital in Los Angeles, CA. She told me her story.

I was in the hospital, wearing a neck brace. I was given medication for pain control, but I wasn't in too much pain. I started throwing up after they gave me morphine. They gave me more morphine and then added in other medications. I kept throwing up and developed a violent headache, the worst I'd ever had. They simply gave me more medication.

The nurses and doctors stopped coming to see me except to give me more medication. I threw up for days. I was neglected and abandoned in that hospital. Being a good patient, I did not want to complain, nor for my husband to complain, at that time or later. The icing on the cake was when I got home and found my own vomit in my neck brace.

I realized after I'd left the hospital that I'd had a side effect or allergic reaction to the morphine.

STEP 2

Check Dosages

Always check dosages. If you notice that a medication dosage has increased, ask why. Be polite, as it may be your mistake, or it may have been ordered by the doctor for a reason. Take notes in the Quick Reference Guide, pages 147, 152.

STEP 3

Check the IV

If the patient is given IV fluids, ask what the IV fluid is for and what the name of it is. Ask the nurse to recheck the label. Write it down in the Quick Reference Guide, page 153. Make sure that everything the patient is connected to is functioning. Trace the IV lines.

But do not under any circumstances take off the IV tubing, turn off feeding tube pumps, change any settings, or do anything to interfere with the equipment. Simply watch, oversee, make notes, and bring anything unusual to the primary nurse's attention.

Write down the answers to your questions in the Daily Progress Notes section. You will recheck each day. If you have other family members in your Family Advocate Team, you will all use each other's notes as a guide.

STEP 4

Check Oxygen, TPN, and Monitors

Check to make sure the oxygen line is actually plugged into the outlet. Trace the line from the mask to its source.

If your loved one is receiving intravenous food (TPN), check the label to make sure it is the correct food. Ask the nurse to compare it with the name on the orders in the patient's chart. Several nurses told me about mistakes made with intravenous food bags because so many of them look alike.

If there are monitors to calculate your loved one's vital signs, such as heartbeat, respirations, and pulse, pay attention to these machines as well. Alarms will sound if something goes wrong. I cannot tell you the number of times I sat with my mother and godmother when the alarm went off and no nurse arrived to solve the problem. I went to the nurses' station and waited for the primary nurse. It is essential that you be proactive.

STEP 5

Check Blood Pressure, Lab, and Test Results

If your loved one has blood drawn, ask for the results. If the vital signs baseline has already been recorded in the Quick Reference Guide, then you only need to note if there is something unusual or abnormal. If so, write this down in the Daily Progress Notes section. Ask the primary nurse what normal test results are and compare. If there is a change or some variation, ask questions.

If the patient goes for an x-ray, ask for the results. Ask what the results mean. Write down every test and result that deviates from the norm. You will be able to compare results with the previous day's results. Watch for inconsistencies. Ask questions.

STEP 6

Check Procedures and Treatments

If your loved one is scheduled for a procedure or treatment, ask the primary nurse what it is and when it will be done. Keep in mind that there can be delays due to emergencies.

> *Be sure the orderly who comes to pick up the patient has the right chart. Recheck the patient's name and date of birth.*
>
> KAREN, RN, WEST HILLS, CA

If you or a member of your Family Advocate Team can be present when these treatments or procedures are taking place, all the better. When the technician arrives, ask what the treatment is or what procedure the patient is scheduled for. Compare notes with the technician. Make sure that they have the correct name of the patient and the correct name of the treatment and/or procedure.

Ask if you can accompany the patient to their treatment or procedure, and wait in the other department's waiting area. Stay with the patient before and after and leave with them.

STEP 7

Get Proactive if the Hospital Doesn't Offer the Patient's Current Medication

Hospital formularies are allowed to carry certain medications and not others, as dictated by their insurance company. Your loved one might be given different medications from what they have been taking at home. These are not medication errors.

If your loved one does not seem to be responding well to the medication provided and you know he or she does well on a certain medication, discuss with the primary care physician the possibility of bringing medication the patient is used to. Then ask your loved one if they would like to have it brought in for them. If it is approved, you will give the medication to the primary nurse.

If your loved one isn't doing well, it might be worth asking the primary nurse or physician what medication the patient is receiving and if there is a possibility of there being a reaction to it. If there is the possibility, it might be worth asking the doctor about switching to a different medication.

If any medications that the patient used to be taking have been withdrawn, ask if there might be withdrawal symptoms.

STEP 8

If You Notice an Error, Talk to the Primary Nurse

If you notice a change in the patient's medication, don't assume the worst right away. Simply pose the question to the primary nurse. You could say, "I noticed that Jim was taking (medication name) for his blood pressure. He didn't get that pill today, and I noticed there was a new blue one. Has there been a change?"

Be nice and polite.

If an error has been made, first go to the primary nurse. Tell them about what occurred and who made the error. Then report it to the nurse supervisor. Call the primary care physician as well. Take notes on what occurred, whom you spoke with, and the times and dates your conversations took place. Record this information in the Daily Progress Notes section.

STEP 9

Monitor the Patient's Diet

Errors can occur with the patient's diet as well. Think about how many patients are in the hospital and how many names the staff has to keep track of. Names can get mixed up and dietary instructions can also be confused.

Make a list of any dietary restrictions for your loved one in the Quick Reference Guide, page 161. If they are to be given a soft diet, check the meal trays that arrive. If the patient has diabetes, check to be sure there are no sugary meals and desserts. If regular snacks are to be provided, check for the regularity and composition of those snacks. Ask the primary nurse if you can bring in snacks, such as healthy alternatives to what is offered in the hospital.

Ask the primary nurse if you can bring meals from home or from a restaurant. Hospital food is not terribly appetizing and this would be a gift to your loved one. Many nurses reported that some patients, if they don't like the food, just won't eat it. But be sure to follow dietary restrictions for the patient.

Notes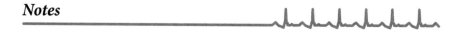

CHAPTER 7

Preventing Infectious Diseases in the Hospital

The number one thing to remember in any hospital setting is to wash your hands. **LOUISE, RN, BOSTON, MA**

THE RISK IS HIGH FOR CONTRACTING A VIRUS or bacteria in the hospital. MRSA, pneumonia, and other hospital-acquired infections are rampant in hospitals. According to the Centers for Disease Control (CDC), there are 1.7 million health care-associated infections every year.

MRSA, methicillin-resistant *Staphylococcus aureus*, is a virulent staph infection that is resistant to many antibiotics. MRSA most often appears as a skin infection, resembling a boil or abscess.

Pneumonia can be deadly and is reported as the most common hospital-acquired infection. It is easily contracted by patients who are on ventilators and who are in the ICU.

According to the American Hospital Association's Quality Center, each year nearly two million patients in the United States get an infection in the hospital. Of those patients, about 90,000 die as a result of their infection. More than 70% of the bacteria that cause hospital-acquired infections are resistant to several antibiotics. Patients infected with drug-resistant infections are likely to require longer hospital stays.

> *Family's Story*
>
> Amelia's father was admitted to the hospital for hip replacement surgery. He was in good health and considered fit. During his recovery from his surgery, he contracted hospital pneumonia. He never left the hospital.

STEP 1

Wash Your Hands

If there are only one or two things you take from this book, take this: *wash your hands, wash your hands, wash your hands.* This is to help prevent the spread of infectious diseases. Every time you enter the patient's room, wash your hands. You may have touched any number of surfaces, such as doorknobs, countertops, or elevator buttons that other visiting families, nurses, doctors, and staff will have touched as well. They may not have washed their hands after visiting sick patients. You don't want to spread what is on your fingers to an already sick patient.

Place a note in the patient's room requesting that people wash their hands or wear disposable gloves to prevent communicable diseases. This issue cannot be emphasized enough.

Ellen, a surgical technician from Los Angeles, CA, said, "I always have a paper towel to use when opening any door in the hospital."

STEP 2

Request a Private Room

You can request a private room. If one is available in the hospital, your loved one will have to pay for it out of pocket.

STEP 3

Ask About Antibiotics

Ask the primary care physician if your loved one will be receiving antibiotics before or after surgery. This is sometimes done to lower the risk of infection.

STEP 4

Use Antibacterial Gel

Place antibacterial gel on the patient's beside table and ask everyone who enters the room to use it. No one should touch the patient without first washing their hands, using antibacterial gel, or wearing a fresh pair of disposable gloves.

In some hospitals, there will be an antibacterial gel dispenser outside the patient's room. Ask everyone to use it.

STEP 5

Avoid Touching Meal Tray Tables

Most all interviewed nurses said, "Do not touch the meal tray table and then touch your loved one." Doctors and nurses place items on that tray table that have been in other sick patient's rooms. Use antibacterial wipes on these tables.

STEP 6

Avoid Using the Patient's Bathroom

Do not use the patient's bathroom. Think about the number of nurses and technicians who enter that bathroom, touch the doorknob, and touch the sink and toilet handle. They have come from other patients' rooms. You do not want to touch something in their bathroom and then touch the patient. The idea alone is enough to make you become obsessive about it.

ABC News reported recently that tens of thousands die each year because of the spread of infectious diseases in hospitals.

STEP 7

Don't Bring in Your Purse, Backpack, or Briefcase

If you carry a purse, backpack, or briefcase, try not to bring it into the patient's room. The bottom of these items has been on more floors and surfaces than you want to remember. You could bring in a disease or bacteria, or you could leave with one and transfer it elsewhere.

STEP 8

Leave Children at Home

Do not bring young children or babies into the hospital if you can help it. Not only are babies prone to crawl on a hospital floor, which is littered with diseases, bacteria, blood, urine, and a host of other unhealthy things, but they also carry germs and are susceptible to germs. Leave them at home if you can.

STEP 9

If You Are Sick, Avoid the Patient

If you are sick, stay away from the hospital. Understandably, you want to see your loved one, but you can transfer diseases to not only your loved one but to other patients as well. If you feel you must visit, then

---

Family's Story

My story: I cringe when I remember bringing my two-year-old daughter into my godmother's hospital room. She crawled on the floor until I noticed a used needle and bloody bandage lying in the corner. I picked her up immediately and never brought her back again. I just didn't know. You may not either. Now you do.

wear an "N95" mask. You can buy one of these at any drugstore, or the hospital may provide one for you.

STEP 10

What to Do if the Nurse or Doctor is Sick

If you see that your loved one's primary nurse is ill, politely ask them to wear a mask. Many nurses I interviewed said that this can be a little tricky, but they all agreed it is absolutely necessary.

The same is true for the doctors. If you notice that the doctor has not washed their hands before touching your loved one, ask politely that they do so, or to put on a fresh pair of gloves. Your request may incite some annoyance. Keep your eye on your goal: to support the best possible medical care for your loved one.

You can pose the request as a soft question: "Doctor, I know this may sound paranoid, but I'm concerned about Jim catching a disease in the hospital. Would you mind washing your hands before touching him?"

STEP 11

Wash Your Hands after Using the Hospital Elevator Buttons

Imagine how many people use the hospital elevator in a day. Doctors, technicians, nurses, visitors, and other staff are all using the buttons in the elevator. This may seem picky and a bit compulsive, but these buttons for the hospital floors are touched by people who have just touched patients who have infectious diseases.

Wash your hands or use antibacterial gel or a wipe after you use the buttons.

Notes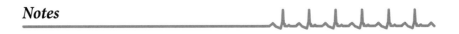

CHAPTER 8

Preventing Fatal Falls

Sometimes I have to resort to using restraints on a patient if I think he might fall out of bed. That can't happen on my watch. **ANONYMOUS, RN, MIAMI, FL**

FATAL FALLS ARE A LEADING CAUSE OF DEATH in hospitals today. You might think only the elderly fall out of bed. Elderly patients are particularly at risk, but so is your loved one if they are recovering from anesthesia or are heavily medicated. If they need to go to the bathroom and a nurse isn't available, offer to help.

Drowsiness is a common side effect of many meds given in the hospital, and special care should be taken to prevent falls and injuries when a patient is drowsy.
KAREN BLANCHARD, MD, SANTA MONICA, CA

STEP 1

Supervise the Patient if They Are a Fall Risk

Patients of all ages and stages of recovery are at risk for falling out of bed. This can be fatal. If the primary nurse and doctor have said the patient is supposed to stay in bed and get out only with assistance, supervise your loved one. You can record information on fall prevention in the Quick Reference Guide, page 161.

Patients can pull out their IVs, try to get out of bed, and become emotionally upset when they are restrained. The hospital nursing staff is not equipped with enough nurses to watch your loved one every minute. They may request a sitter if your loved one is a danger to himself or to others.

Amy, a registered nurse from Oakland, CA, said this: "We have an increasing population of confused patients. People are living longer. Everyone is so afraid that confused patients will pull out their lines or get out of bed and fall. We have liability. If a family member is there, I don't have to worry about restraining them."

If your loved one is confined to bed, you can help them stay there. Members of your Family Advocate Team must all be aware of this, and one of you must be with the patient at all times. In the Daily Progress Notes, write down the schedule for members of your Family Advocate Team who will sit with your loved one.

STEP 2

Hire a Sitter, Companion, or Private Duty Nurse

You can hire a private duty nurse, companion, or sitter to keep your loved one in bed. Review Step 12 in Chapter 3 for more information on these caregivers.

STEP 3

Prevent the Need for Patient Restraints

Several nurses I spoke to admitted using physical restraints on some patients, even if they didn't want to, because they just couldn't leave their patient at risk.

A number of nurses reported that the use of any kind of restraint upsets family members. Seeing your loved one with straps on their ankles and wrists might be frightening. Know that it is for good reason and is not being done out of cruelty.

You can prevent the need for restraints if you sit with your loved one and prevent them from pulling out IV lines and prevent them from falling.

Family's Story

Christy's father went out to dinner, became disoriented on the drive home, and had a car accident. He ended up in a hospital outside of New York. He had suffered a stroke and a hip fracture.

My sister and I lived out of state. My dad was there so long that he developed hospital psychosis and became agitated at night. The nurses put him into restraints, which upset him further. They left meal trays in his room which he never got around to eating before someone else picked them up.

This hospital was terribly understaffed. After his first surgery, he went downhill fast. When I visited him, he tried to pull out the screws that held pins in his leg. He was completely disoriented. The hospital said they couldn't offer a sitter because he wasn't a danger to himself or others. His room was far away from the nurses' station. He was unable to press the button when he needed their help. There were mix-ups in his treatment, such as when the respiratory therapist wasn't called and the nurse thought he had been called.

There was total miscommunication. If I hadn't been there, he would have died. I came back a week later to find my dad's tooth broken. I asked the nurse about this. She said it must have occurred in his accident. I knew my father's tooth was intact the last time I'd been there. I knew he had fallen.

Some nurses and key hospital officials were angels; other nurses didn't care. Thank God my sister and I got him out of there.

Notes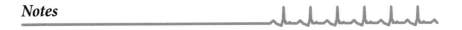

CHAPTER 9

Language Barriers and Cultural Issues

If you're from a different culture, have a family member who is more familiar with our customs be an interface.

ANGELA, RN, PHILADELPHIA, PA

STEP 1

Inform Medical Staff About Cultural Preferences

Some cultures have preferences regarding touching and caring for the patient. They may also have preferences about foods and treatments. Be sure to alert your loved one's primary nurse to any of these preferences and guidelines. The nurse may not know unless you provide the information. A section at the back of this book, page 161, is provided for you to record notes on cultural preferences and issues. Use this page so that information will be readily available to all members of the Family Advocate Team, as well as to private duty nurses, sitters, and companions.

STEP 2

If the Patient Doesn't Speak English, Translate

Most doctors and nurses I interviewed were emphatic about having someone translate for the patient if the patient doesn't speak English. A number of other nurses told me stories about patients who did not speak

Nurse's Story

Jackie, a registered nurse from Stanton, CA, said this:

I had a patient who only spoke Spanish. I speak English. He had chest pains. I could only ask basic questions. His daughter came to me and said, "You should learn to speak Spanish." I can't be expected to be fluent in several different languages. This situation with my patient could have compromised his care.

English, and because of this, their care could have been compromised. If your loved one cannot speak English, you can help by translating during doctor visits and meetings with the primary nurse.

STEP 3

Be Sure Someone is There to Translate

If you won't be there to do the translating, the nurse will find a hospital translator. However, most hospitals have only one translator for the entire hospital. Many use phone-based translation service provided by AT&T, but many interviewed nurses said that this service, although very helpful, is time consuming and cumbersome. Time may be of the essence for your loved one.

> *Participate in your loved one's care. With non-English-speaking patients, be at the bedside and choose one in your family who speaks English.*
>
> CHERYL, RN,
> FOUNTAIN VALLEY, CA

Keep in mind that doctors and nurses cannot treat a patient if they cannot understand them.

A number of nurses did not like relying on the "by-phone" translation services, because they could not be sure that the interpreter was explaining the information correctly to the patient. Some nurses refused to use them for fear of some vital piece of information being missed or left out.

STEP 4

If It's an Emergency, Translate for the Patient

If an interpreter is not available, and the patient is in an emergency situation, do not belabor the necessity for having a translator from the hospital. Translate yourself or find someone who will translate for you.

> *Remember:*
> *This is time limited.*
> *This is worth your time right now.*
> *You could save a life.*

STEP 5

Bring in Food for Your Loved One

Bringing in food from the outside for patients of a different culture is also helpful. Sometimes meals from our culture are not suitable for certain patients. Ask the primary care nurse what you can bring. Write down these dietary alternatives and cultural preferences in the Quick Reference Guide, page 161.

Notes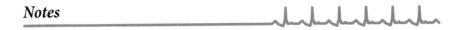

CHAPTER 10

Special Attention Required on Routine Medical and Surgical Floors

A family member's involvement as advocate is more important on other floors, because there is not as much coverage with nurses. In the ICU, it is one nurse to two patients. Family members are patients' best advocates.

ROBERT ADAIR, MD, SANTA MONICA, CA

IF YOUR LOVED ONE IS A PATIENT on any floor except for the ICU, you will need to be extra vigilant with all the steps outlined in this book. Nurses on these floors may be less trained, have more patients to care for, have less time, and have more paperwork. Sometimes nurse-to-patient ratios on these floors can be as low as 1:10.

STEP 1

Initiate a Relationship with the New Nurse

The entire process with primary nurses begins again when your loved one is transferred to another floor. Go back to Chapter 3, "The Primary Nurse", and reread it. Keep notes on the patient's new hospital floor in the Quick Reference Guide, page 162. Each step is so important and can be even more important on other floors, because there may be fewer nurses to tend to patients. For example, your loved one may press the buzzer and it may take much longer for the nurse to arrive. You and your loved one might spend more time waiting for almost everything on these floors. This is not because the nurses don't care, but because they are caring for more patients and doing more paperwork.

The earlier steps about schmoozing the primary nurse are even more important on these floors.

Remember:

1. Establish a relationship with the new primary nurses.

2. Chat informally with each of them.

3. Humanize the patient.

4. Offer to help with patient care.

5. Express appreciation for the nurses' care of the patient.

STEP 2

Pay Close Attention

If your loved one is on any floor other than ICU, pay close attention. Since nurse-to-patient ratios go down on these floors, there are more chances for errors to occur. This means that you must monitor every transaction more closely.

STEP 3

Monitor Medications, Tests, and Treatments More Carefully

Be aware that while your loved one is a patient on a routine medical or surgical floor, you and your Family Advocate Team will need to be with the patient more regularly and monitor medications, treatments, and procedures more carefully. You will need to be more proactive on

Family's Story

Bill Brighton was admitted to the hospital. He'd had two major heart attacks and was recovering in the ICU. His wife, Rachel, walked in one morning to find her husband's arms waving in the air and his face turning quite red. He had a tracheotomy and was on a ventilator. The respiratory therapist's back was turned. When Rachel saw her husband's plight, she screamed, "He can't breathe."

It turned out that the respiratory therapist had cleaned Bill's trach tube and had accidentally left the plug in. Bill, in fact, could not breathe. Imagine what would have happened if Rachel had not walked in at that moment. Rachel and her sons brought the incident to the attention of the cardiologist, the primary nurse, and the nurse supervisor. Bill Brighton had no further incidents and was discharged from the hospital alive and well.

these floors, especially at night, on holidays and weekends, and during summer months. Review the steps in Chapter 6, "Preventing Medical Error."

STEP 4

Prevent the Spread of Infectious Diseases

Because the number of patients increases on these floors, the possibility for the spread of infectious diseases increases. Oversee that doctors, nurses, and technicians wash their hands or wear a fresh pair of disposable gloves before touching your loved one. Put a sign above the patient's bed requesting that all who enter the room wash their hands. Keep antibacterial gel handy next to the patient's bed. Be vigilant. Review the steps in Chapter 7 on preventing infectious diseases.

If your loved one has a roommate, this means double the number of people who enter your loved one's room. You don't know where they have been, and you don't know what is on their hands or on the bottom of their purses, backpacks, clipboards, and briefcases.

You can inform them of the nature of hospital-acquired infection. This situation can be delicate, but if you ask nicely and tell visitors that your loved one's immune system is compromised and that you are simply looking out for the patient, they most likely will understand.

Remember:
This is time limited.
This is worth your time right now.
You could save a life.

STEP 5

What to Do if the Patient Has a Problem Roommate

Roommates can be a blessing for some patients and a curse for others. If your loved one has a roommate with problems that interfere with necessary rest and recovery, ask your loved one if they would like to change rooms. This is a simple procedure. Find the charge nurse or nurse supervisor on the floor, explain the situation, and ask for a room change.

STEP 6

Monitor Meals

Because there may be two to three patients to a room, monitor the diet for your loved one. Check to see that the patient is receiving the diet that the doctor has ordered. See that they are eating their meals. They may need assistance. You can help.

Notes

Notes

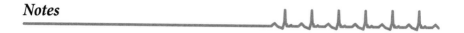

CHAPTER 11

If You Live Out of Town

It is very difficult to deal with family from out of town. Sometimes nurses don't even talk to out-of-town family members unless there is some change in the condition of the patient. And they may only talk to them if they are the Responsible Party, or have power of attorney.

LISA, NURSE SUPERVISOR, DETROIT, MI

What to Do If You Need to Travel to Visit Your Loved One

STEP 1

Get Assistance with Housing and Hotels

If you live out of town and your loved one has a dire medical crisis, try to find a way to get there. Not every hospital has an in-house social worker, but call and ask. If it does, call the hospital social worker and ask if there are local hotels that offer discounted rates for family members with loved ones in the hospital. Ask the social worker if the hospital has any housing for out-of-town family members.

STEP 2

Ask the Airlines for Reduced Rates

If you plan to fly to visit your loved one, ask the airlines if they give a reduced rate for medical emergencies. Many do. Each time I reserved my flight to visit my mother in the hospital in Colorado, I told the airlines that my mother was in the ICU and I asked if they could give me a reduced rate. They did each time.

Call the hospital social worker and ask if there are any transportation services to help you once you have arrived.

STEP 3

Reread Chapters 2 (The Basics of Being an Advocate), 3 (The Primary Nurse), 4 (The Doctors), and 5 (The Importance of Research)

Once you arrive at your loved one's hospital, reread chapters 2–5 and follow each of the steps.

STEP 4

Contact Relatives and Friends

You will need to gather support once you arrive in the city where your loved one is hospitalized. Contact relatives and friends and talk to them about the patient and the patient's condition. Ask your loved one if they want any of these people to visit.

STEP 5

Use the Social Worker

Once you have secured housing and transportation, contact the hospital social worker if you have not already done so (see Chapter 13, "Hospital Social Workers").

If need be, ask about legal services for DNR, Power of Attorney, etc.

If You Can't Travel to Visit Your Loved One

STEP 1

Call the Hospital

Call the hospital where your loved one is a patient and ask what floor the patient is on. Call the floor and ask for the nurses' station. Ask for the patient's primary nurse. If the primary nurse isn't available, ask for the charge nurse. Ask the charge nurse for the primary nurse's name and direct phone number. Write it down in the Quick Reference Guide, page 150.

STEP 2

Introduce Yourself to the Primary Nurse

Introduce yourself to the primary nurse and ask what the diagnosis, treatment plan, and prognosis are for the patient. Write everything down in the Quick Reference Guide.

STEP 3

Ask the Primary Nurse for the Name of the Primary Care Physician

Ask who the primary care physician is. Write down their name and direct phone number in the Quick Reference Guide. Ask the primary nurse to leave a note in the patient's chart for the doctor to call you when they arrive. Ask what time that doctor does rounds. Stay near the phone at that time. If you don't hear from the doctor, make another call.

STEP 4

Ask Questions

When you speak to the doctor, go through all the steps in Chapter 4 ("The Doctors"). But since you are out of town, you will be asking a few more questions. After asking all the sample questions on page 50, then ask these:

1. Since I'm out of town, how can I reach you directly if I have questions?

2. Will you be in town to take care of my loved one, or are you going on vacation?

3. If you are not on call, which doctor do I contact? What is his or her name and phone number?

4. Would you suggest that I hire a sitter to be with my loved one during the day or at night? If so, how would I find one?

5. Would you suggest I fly out to be there?

6. When are the procedures, treatments, or operation scheduled?

List planned procedures, treatments, etc. in the Quick Reference Guide. Call on that day to ask how the procedures or operation went.

STEP 5

Establish a Relationship with the Nurse

There may be a different primary nurse on shift each day and night when you call. Review all the steps about establishing a relationship with each one. Write down the nurses' names and the dates you spoke with them in the Daily Progress Notes. Take notes on the conversations.

STEP 6

Consider Hiring a Private Duty Nurse, Sitter, or Companion

If you don't have a couple of family members or good friends in town to help you, you might consider hiring a private duty nurse, sitter, or companion to help oversee and monitor your loved one's care. This is

Family's Story

Frank's father was in the emergency room in another state, having suffered a heart attack. Frank's stepmother told him the basics of his father's condition. But Frank wanted to speak directly to the doctors and his father's primary nurse. Since he didn't know what to do, he simply sat back and waited to hear further reports from his stepmother.

After I realized how helpless he felt because of not being able to speak to the doctor or even to his father, I suggested that he could in fact reach the doctor, the primary nurse, and his father. I told him, "You don't have to just sit back and wait. Here's how you do it." I outlined the steps for him, as follows:

1. Call the nurses' station in the ER. Ask for your father's primary nurse. If they are not available, get their name, write it down, and call back. Keep calling.

2. When you reach the primary nurse, ask how your father is, what his current diagnosis is, what the treatment plan is, and ask who the primary physician is—that's the main doctor who is taking care of him. Write down his or her name. Ask how they can be reached.

The doctor just happened to be there when Frank called. He went through two very similar conversations with the primary nurse and the doctor. He gained a sense of what was going on and what was being done for his father.

Frank was then able to speak to his father in the ER. It made his father feel better too. Being alone in the ER is no fun. It's isolating and frightening. Frank felt better having been proactive instead of waiting for his stepmother to phone him with information. He let the doctor and primary nurse know that he was concerned and involved.

Remember what the doctors and nurses have said: "Patients with involved family members get better care."

Frank's dad later told him that he felt comforted after speaking with him on the phone.

especially important at night, on weekends, on holidays, and during summer months.

Ask the patient's primary nurse, the hospital social worker, or the hospital patient advocate (if they have one) for referrals.

Send a copy of this book to the person you hire. Ask them to read it and discuss pertinent chapters with them. Ask them to take notes in the Daily Progress Notes section. Speak to them daily about your loved one's progress.

> *Being involved gets more attention. Call regularly. Get a family member or friend who lives in town to go see the patient. The staff needs to know someone is checking up on the patient. If no one ever inquires, the patient might get ignored.*
>
> MARILYN, RN,
> LAKEWOOD, CA

STEP 7

Call to Check In

Call the nurses' station each day and find out who the primary nurse is for your loved one. When you speak to them, ask how your loved one is doing. This serves two purposes: you are letting them know that you are involved, and you will also get accurate information about the status of your loved one.

STEP 8

Call the Patient

Telephone the patient every day, depending on how alert and well they are. If your loved one doesn't feel well, call the primary nurse instead. Ask them to tell your loved one that you called to check in to see how they are doing. Take notes.

Here are some sample questions to ask your loved one:

1. How are you feeling today?

2. Has anything changed since yesterday?

3. Are you able to reach the nurse for pain medication and other needs? If they say no, consider hiring a sitter or enlisting a friend or family member to check in on your loved one. There is nothing worse than being alone in the hospital and waiting for pain medication and no one comes or you can't reach the call button.

4. Is your roommate OK? Is he or she quiet? Is he or she receiving a lot of visitors? If the answer is yes to the latter, ask your loved one if they would like to switch rooms. Explain that you can facilitate that. Then call the charge nurse on the floor, explain the situation, and ask if your loved one can be moved to another room.

5. Each day ask about your loved one's improvement. If there is none, or if there are setbacks, ask what your loved one's symptoms are and write them down in the Daily Progress Notes section at the back of this book. Call the patient's primary nurse and physician to discuss the situation with the two of them.

STEP 9

Enlist a Friend or Family Member

Ask a friend or family member who lives in town to visit your loved one every day. Ask them to call or email you with reports. Discuss the patient's condition. Compare notes on conversations with the patient's doctors and nurses. Share your observations of the patient's health status. If your friend or family member has impressions of your loved one's health status that differ from your own, make notes and call the doctor and primary nurse.

Send your friend or family member a copy of this book. Schedule a time for a phone conversation to go over pertinent chapters. Ask them to take notes in the Quick Reference Guide and Daily Progress Notes sections.

> ### Nurse's Story
> Kathy, an RN in Seattle, WA, said,
>
> *My mother was in a hospital in another state. I talked to my mom on the phone and she sounded fine. I'd enlisted help from my niece, who went and visited her the next day. My mother didn't recognize her. I called the charge nurse and reported the experience and asked if maybe my mom was overmedicated or if she'd had a stroke.*

STEP 10

Send Cookies or Candy to the Primary Nurses

When you live out of town, it is especially important to make an impression on the patient's primary nurses and to express appreciation for all they are doing for your loved one. Send a basket of cookies/candy with the primary nurses' names on the card, complete with the hospital floor and name of the unit. Ask the food company if they can staple the card to the basket of cookies so the nurses will know your loved one's family sent them. You don't want that card getting lost or tossed. You want them to remember you and your loved one.

Notes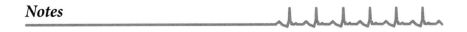

Notes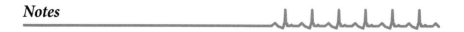

CHAPTER 12

How to Support and Comfort Your Loved One

Don't come into the patient's room with your own agenda.
Ask how the patient is. Let the patient set the pace for the
interaction.

LINDA VENTURA, SOCIAL WORKER, UCLA, LOS ANGELES, CA

STEP 1

Focus on the Patient

Put your own anxiety aside when visiting your loved one. They are frightened and want to know that everything is going to be all right. Reassure them. Explain that you are involved in their care and will help to oversee it. A few words to let them know that they are going to get better and that you will do everything you can to make sure they are comfortable will go a long way. As you read through this chapter and as you discuss with your loved one some of the things that would increase their comfort, take notes. Keep your notes in the section provided in the Quick Reference Guide, pages 159, 160. Make sure that all members of the Family Advocate Team have access to these notes.

STEP 2

Bring the Outside World into the Hospital

All families, doctors, and nurses I interviewed said that the more you can do to bring the outside world into the hospital room, the better the patient will feel. Translation? The faster the recovery.

Ask the primary nurse if you can bring in blankets and cozy comforters, pillows, pajamas, and photos to put on the bulletin board or in a frame next to the bed. If an MP3 player, DVD player, stuffed animal, or family photos are desired by the patient, and approved by the primary nurse, bring them in, even if your loved one is only in the hospital for a short stay.

> *Sit with the patient for companionship; whatever your loved one would want to make them feel more at home. Ask if you can bring in their comfortable sheets or pillowcase. If the patient is religious, bring in prayers on tape.*
> CAROL, RN, PASADENA, CA

Hospitals are not homey, comfortable places, and anything you can bring in from home and the outside world will add to your loved one's peace of mind. Personal hygiene items, such as toothbrush, toothpaste, hairbrush, razor, and shampoo, are all nice touches. Some hospitals have barber/beautician in-house services.

Bring in magazines, newspapers, and music. There are many studies that show that music has healing properties. Generally, hospitals provide very small radios only at the patient's bedside. They don't sound great and may not play what your loved one wants to hear. Bring a CD player with headphones so other patients won't be disturbed.

One family member, John, made audiotapes of his father's favorite songs and brought them into the hospital.

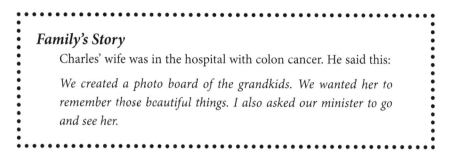

Family's Story

Charles' wife was in the hospital with colon cancer. He said this:

We created a photo board of the grandkids. We wanted her to remember those beautiful things. I also asked our minister to go and see her.

STEP 3

Include the Patient in the Conversation

If the patient is alert, it is important that they be a part of their treatment. Keep your loved one in the loop of communication with everyone. There is nothing worse than doctors, nurses, or visitors talking over the patient as if he were not there. You want to help your loved one feel empowered, and talking over him will only create a sense of helplessness and frustration.

STEP 4

Be Positive About the Patient's Recovery

Your loved one will take the cue from you and other family members about their health and prognosis. Be positive and supportive. Doctors and nurses all said that patients recover more quickly if their family and friends have positive attitudes.

STEP 5

Respect the Patient

Ask the patient what they need. Do they want to talk or not? Do they want privacy? Do they want visitors, and if so, who? Phone calls?

Don't talk on your cell phone in front of the patient.

If there are other visitors in the room, don't have conversations with those visitors that don't involve the patient.

STEP 6

Listen to the Patient

A social worker from a major hospital in Los Angeles, CA, said, "Allow them (the patient) to process their feelings. Expression of emotion is healing. Don't try to fix it." She explained that patients tell her that families want their loved ones to feel better. Allow your loved one to feel bad and allow them to cry. You can cry too.

STEP 7

Be Aware the Patient Can Hear You

Many nurses told me that the patient can still hear you even if he or she is asleep or not alert. Be careful about discussing a grim prognosis in front of your loved one. Step outside the room to have this type of conversation.

STEP 8

Keep Stress Away from the Patient

If you are upset, leave it outside the patient's room. Many nurses reported that too often family members will enter the room upset and then upset the patient. Stress is never helpful for a patient's recovery.

STEP 9

Ask for Spiritual Help

Ask the patient if they would like their minister, chaplain, deacon, rabbi, etc., to visit. Often, hospitals will have their own deacons or religious professionals. You can always request their services as well.

STEP 10

Bring in Meals from Home

Ask the primary nurse if you can bring in meals from home. This is a nice touch for some patients and makes them feel more comfortable. This is also helpful for patients from other cultures who might not eat if offered food from our culture. If the patient isn't allowed to eat, don't bring in food and eat in front of them.

STEP 11

Ask the Patient if They Want to Be Touched

First ask the primary nurse if lotion and massage are OK. If so, then ask the patient if they would like you to massage their hands, feet, or back. Bring in lotion. Touch can enhance healing and help patients feel less alone. Many nurses reported that patients need to be touched.

> *Family's Story*
>
> My story: I massaged my mom's feet and hands regularly. It seemed to bring her comfort in the midst of a terrible situation. She was on full life support and there wasn't much else we could do.

STEP 12

Keep Your Loved One Mentally Stimulated

TV is the common babysitter in the hospital. You can provide input that may be more personally meaningful, stimulating, and interesting to the patient. Keep them abreast of what is going on in the news or in your town. Report news about family, friends, and business associates. Ask family, friends, and associates to write get well cards and send them to the hospital.

Phone calls are fine, but try to keep them to a minimum. You can ask the primary nurse for help. The patient needs rest, and if there is a roommate, the roommate needs rest too.

STEP 13

Call the Patient's Family and Employer

Offer to call the patient's family, friends, and place of employment to tell them about your loved one's hospitalization.

My mom was in the hospital. She was very agitated, screaming. All these people were walking in. It was upsetting her. I asked the primary nurse if I could put up a sign for people not to come in.

Also, if you hear drawers slamming and it disturbs the patient, ask nicely, "Do you mind?" It's a matter of educating the staff too. Dispense your knowledge kindly and gently.

ELLEN, SURGICAL TECHNICIAN, LOS ANGELES, CA

STEP 14

Ask About Pets at Home

Ask if the patient has a dog or cat at home that you or another family member or friend can take care of while they are hospitalized.

STEP 15

Control Noise

Noise can affect sleep and recovery. If there is a lot of noise at the nurses' station, ask the primary nurse if it is permissible to shut the patient's door. If the roommate's phone is constantly ringing, talk to the primary nurse about it.

STEP 16

Keep Visitors to a Minimum

Visitors are great, but more is not the merrier. Depending on the illness or injury of the patient, keep visitors to a minimum in the room. Too many can overwhelm the patient. Take turns. Ask the visitors if they would mind waiting until one or two other visitors leave.

Countless hospital RNs expressed exasperation about there being too many visitors in the patient's room. Since you are the point person, you are in charge of this. You can enlist the primary nurse's help at any time, because their goal is the same as yours: the well-being and recovery of their patient.

Nurses offered many suggestions. Here is what most of them said:

1. Do not have more than two people in the hospital room at any one time. If a visitor is waiting to see the patient, one visitor should volunteer to leave so another can come in.

2. It is intrusive for a number of visitors to enter the room all at once, especially if the nurse needs to give a bath, do a procedure, or check the patient's vital signs. If the nurse enters, ask whether you and the other visitors should leave. Many procedures are private.

3. The patient needs to sleep! Allow time for rest and recuperation. Do not stay and have a party in the patient's room.

4. Do not talk to one another over the patient. Involve them in the conversation. If the patient is tired, leave the room.

5. If your loved one has a roommate, be considerate and do not disturb the roommate's rest.

STEP 17

How to Handle a Problem Roommate

If a roommate has become a problem for your loved one, you can talk to the charge nurse or nurse supervisor about a room change.

My godmother, Martha, had a roommate with dementia who stood over her and yelled in the middle of the night. Needless to say, this scared Martha very badly. At 81, she didn't need that. I spoke to the nurse supervisor and the change was made the next morning.

STEP 18

How to Spot Hospital Psychosis

Hospital psychosis can occur with patients who have been in the hospital for a while. They become disoriented and can become delusional. If you notice signs of hallucinations, strange speech, or that your loved one is acting odd, contact the primary nurse immediately. Tell them everything you have observed. Show the nurse your notes documented in this book.

Remember:
Your goal is to support the
best possible medical care
for your loved one.

STEP 19

Defuse Frustration Among Family Members

Frustrations among family members are bound to flare up from time to time. It's understandable to be upset about your loved one's health. All interviewed nurses said this: "I hate to see family members fighting in front of the patient."

Arguing in front of the patient is not only detrimental to their well-being, but can also be detrimental to recovery. They will feel stressed if you create conflict in front of them. Take any heated discussions outside the patient's room. Find a third party, deacon, other religious professional, or social worker in the hospital to help you sort out any disagreement regarding patient care.

Notes

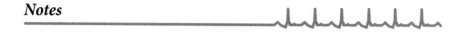

Notes

CHAPTER 13

Hospital Social Workers

If the hospital has a social worker, use them. Ask them for resources, for support. **JANET, RN, PLEASANTON, CA**

MANY HOSPITALS HAVE IN-HOUSE SOCIAL WORKERS. They can be a wonderful support for family members and patients. They are counselors as well as resource people, and can provide emotional support, offer resources for coping, provide resources for hotels and housing, and can lead you in directions for research and family member support groups.

Some interviewed hospital social workers said they would be willing to intervene on a patient's behalf if the family is having trouble reaching a doctor. Social workers in some hospitals will even help you find movie rentals, video game rentals, art supply rentals, etc.

STEP 1

How to Find the Hospital Social Worker

Simply ask the primary nurse whether the hospital has a social worker. A hospital social worker may even come into the patient's room and make an introduction. Ask for a couple of their business cards. Keep one for yourself and give one to your loved one. List their name and contact information in the Quick Reference Guide, page 158.

STEP 2

What to Do if the Hospital Doesn't Have a Social Worker

Ask the primary nurse for someone who can perform some of the duties of a social worker. Some hospitals have patient advocates. If not, then perhaps an in-house religious professional can fulfill part of that role.

Sometimes a nurse supervisor or case manager can help you with other resources in or out of the hospital. Some hospitals consider all their primary nurses to be advocates for their patients.

> *There are social workers in hospitals. Many people think they are there only for poor people and that isn't true. Social workers are full of resources to help familiarize you with the disease (illness or injury) or to familiarize you with the area if you're from out of town.*
>
> RACHEL, RN,
> PORTLAND, OR

STEP 3

Enlist the Social Worker in Supporting the Patient

It is stressful to be a patient in the hospital. If your loved one appears emotionally stressed or depressed, or if you have noticed signs of hospital psychosis, ask the primary nurse for the social worker's phone number and ask them to pay a visit to the patient. Support is essential for the patient who may simply want to talk or may want help in expressing needs to family members.

STEP 4

Enlist the Social Worker to Help Reduce Family Stress

Hospital social workers can also help you and other family members deal with any differing opinions about your loved one's care or help ease family frustrations. That is what they are there for.

STEP 5

Ask the Social Worker for Resources

Hospital social workers can help you plan ahead if you are traveling into town to visit your loved one. They can help you find reduced-cost housing or housing connected with the hospital. They can help with transportation resources. And they can steer you in the direction of information about your loved one's disease, illness, or injury.

Notes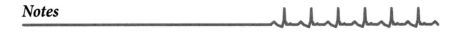

CHAPTER 14

Considering a Different Hospital

Rural hospitals tend to have fewer nurses to care for patients. Teaching hospitals tend to have broader areas of expertise in certain areas because of specialized research they do there.

ANONYMOUS MD, BALTIMORE, MD

IF YOUR LOVED ONE LIVES IN A RURAL AREA and the hospital there does not have a specialty that matches the patient's illness or injury, or if it lacks the specialties the patient needs, consider a transfer to another hospital, either a teaching hospital or a hospital in a metropolitan area. According to Perry A. Henderson, MD, Professor Emeritus, University of Wisconsin Medical School, Madison, WI, "A greater number of physicians elect to practice in urban areas, leaving a physician shortage in rural areas."

If your loved one's condition isn't improving, start asking questions. Should a move be considered to a teaching hospital that specializes in the patient's condition?

If you are considering transferring the patient to a different hospital, there is space for your research and notes in the Quick Reference Guide, page 165. You can take the following steps to help you make a decision:

STEP 1

Call the Patient's Family Physician

If you're considering a transfer to a different hospital, ask your loved one's physician for their opinion on this idea. It's OK to page the doctor if you need to.

STEP 2

Evaluate the Alternative Hospitals

Here are a few ideas to help evaluate hospitals you may be considering.

1. Research hospitals online (www.healthgrades.com).

2. Find out if the hospital is accredited by the Joint Commission (www.jointcommission.org).

3. Find out if the hospital is a Magnet facility. Go to www. nursingworld.org to find out. ["Magnet" status is awarded by the American Nurses Credentialing Center (ANCC)].

4. Ask about nurse-to-patient ratios. Call the hospital directly and ask.

5. Keep in mind that asking about fatality rates will not get you very far. Fatality rates can depend on the illness or injury, age, and health status of the patient, as well as on a host of other variables.

6. Ask if the hospital regularly performs the particular surgery your loved one needs.

7. Ask if the specialist or surgeon at the hospital you are considering is board-certified in his or her specialty.

8. Does your loved one's primary physician recommend or support a move to the hospital you are considering?

9. Does the hospitalist, attending doctor, or other physician recommend or support a move?

10. Is your loved one stabilized?

Family's Story

My story: My mother was admitted to a community hospital when she had acute pancreatitis. Three months into her stay, she took a turn for the worse. I wish I had known that community hospitals may not have physicians who specialize in specific diseases and may not have the experience with specific cases that physicians in teaching hospitals or major city hospitals have. If I'd known that either of these can offer a broader spectrum of care, and/or more experience in certain illnesses, I would have done the research and asked that she be transferred. I just didn't know.

Notes

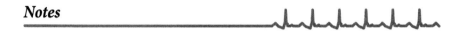

CHAPTER 15

HIPAA Laws, Advance Directives, Power of Attorney, Living Will, and DNR

What we see is that good estate planning makes good sense.

KATHERINE BULTMAN, SOCIAL WORKER,
SAINT JOHN'S MEDICAL CENTER, SANTA MONICA, CA

HIPAA Privacy Rules

HIPAA (Health Insurance Portability and Accountability Act of 1996) maintains confidentiality of your health status and prevents medical professionals from divulging any information about your loved one to anyone who calls or visits, except in certain instances. Some hospitals won't even divulge whether you are a patient there. This law is for good reason, but it can hamper communication with loved ones who call or show up to speak to the doctors and nurses.

Some hospitals may assign a password so family members can call for information about their loved one.

According to the American Hospital Association, HIPAA is a set of national standards for the protection of certain health information. It assures that individuals' health information is properly protected while allowing the flow of health information needed to provide and promote high quality health care and to protect the public's health and well-being.

HIPAA permits important uses of information, while protecting the privacy of people who seek medical care. This rule protects confidentiality and security of health data through setting and enforcing standards.

> ### Nurse's Story
>
> Cheryl, an RN from Fountain Valley, CA, said, "A woman called the nurses' station and said, 'I don't want to bother (patient name). Did she have a boy or girl?' I didn't tell her. The caller kept asking me questions and I said, 'I can't share that information.'
>
> "The caller finally said, 'When her boyfriend goes out of the room, please give (patient name) this message—tell her Amanda is thinking of her.' I waited until the patient's boyfriend left the room and told her what the caller had said. The patient looked horrified. She said, 'That's my boyfriend's ex-girlfriend.'"

Advance Directive

An advance directive, according to the American Hospital Association, is a document written in advance of serious illness. It states your loved one's choices for health care or names someone to make those choices if your loved one becomes unable to do this.

Bring your loved one's advance directive with you to the hospital. Make sure it gets into the patient's chart. Katherine Bultman, a social worker at St. John's Medical Center in Santa Monica, CA, said, "Bringing the advance directive with you is beneficial so we know whom to talk to if the patient can't talk themselves. It's mainly for doctors and nurses so they know whom to talk to when a decision needs to be made."

There is space in the Quick Reference Guide, page 166, to list information on advance directives and other legal documents.

Living Will

A living will, according to the American Hospital Association, is a document in which your loved one stipulates the kind of life-prolonging medical care they want if they become terminally ill, permanently unconscious, or are in a vegetative state and are unable to make their own decisions.

Durable Power of Attorney for Health Care

A Durable Power of Attorney for Health Care, according to the American Hospital Association, is another kind of advance directive. It is a signed, dated, and witnessed document naming another person to make medical decisions for your loved one if they are unable to.

Every interviewed nurse emphasized the importance of every patient having this document with them.

DNR (Do Not Resuscitate)

DNR means Do Not Resuscitate. This means "a medical refrain from resuscitation" if a patient's heart stops beating, according to the American Hospital Association.

Karen Blanchard, MD, had this to say about the resuscitation issue: "Families often have a hard time discussing end-of-life issues and this can lead to treatment that the patient would not have wanted, or inappropriate treatment that would prolong the patient's death rather than prolonging their life.

"A person's right to decide for himself what would constitute living a good life does not end when he or she is no longer able to communicate. Physicians need the patient's guidance, and often the patient's loved ones can provide that perspective."

The optimal situation is if the patient has previously executed the documents mentioned in this chapter. If documents have not been executed, consider executing them as soon as possible. At least initiate a discussion with your loved one about what they would want should they ever be in a precarious health situation in the hospital. No son, daughter, or spouse wants to make decisions for a loved one if these difficult issues have not been addressed.

Notes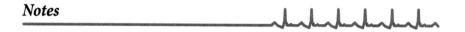

CHAPTER 16

How to Take Care of You

Treat your energy like a bank account. If you use too much, you will deplete it and you'll have to put more in.

DAVID WELLISCH, PHD, CHIEF PSYCHOLOGIST, ADULT DIVISION, DAVID GEFFEN SCHOOL OF MEDICINE, UCLA, LOS ANGELES, CA

ACTING AS YOUR LOVED ONE'S ADVOCATE is a demanding and time-consuming job. It can easily consume you, as it did me when I was caring for my hospitalized mother and godmother. I'd become intensely involved in their care, largely because of my fear of the unknown. Once I started educating myself, I started to relax.

But at first, with both of them, I reacted with shock and then panic about whether they would make it out of the hospital alive. I eventually learned how to moderate my emotional investment in their medical care.

You may have children, a spouse, a job, and other responsibilities. Try to maintain those as best you can. Not only for your own well-being, but for that of your loved one as well. They don't need a nervous advocate at their bedside. They need you to take care of yourself.

There is a section in the Quick Reference Guide, page 167, to guide you.

STEP 1

Make Time for Yourself

You have a life. Part of your life will be taken up with being involved with your loved one and their nurses and doctors. But keep in mind that the best caregivers are the people who also give to themselves. Take time for yourself, away from the hospital and from your other obligations. Do things you enjoy. Just because your loved one is suffering doesn't mean you have to immerse yourself in their suffering all day long, every day.

Take walks, even if you only walk around the hospital. Getting outside of the hospital helps you reorient yourself to the normal world. There is nothing normal about the inside of a hospital.

Go to a movie, read a book, or do something fun with your family and friends.

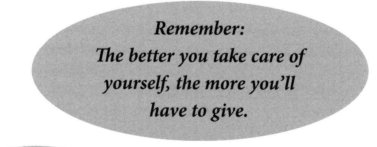

Remember:
The better you take care of
yourself, the more you'll
have to give.

 STEP 2

Enlist the Help of Others

When you start to notice signs of becoming overwhelmed, try to catch it right away and ask for help from friends or family. Ask them to visit the patient for a day or two so that you can take a break. Telephone your loved one that day instead.

If you can afford it, hire a private duty nurse, sitter, companion, or nurse's aide to sit with your loved one so you can get away from the hospital. Give them this book and written instructions for anything you would like done.

STEP 3

Stay Connected to the Outside World

Try to stay connected to the outside world. Just as your loved one will get insulated in the hospital, you might too. Read the newspaper, listen to the radio, or watch TV. It is just as important for you as it is for your loved one.

Exercise is a great stress reliever. If you already exercise, try to stay on your regular routine. If you cannot, take regular walks outdoors to help your body and clear your mind.

If you are in school, stay in school. Study for your classes. Maintain as much of a regular routine as you can. Of course there will be modifications, sometimes major ones, but try to hold onto the structure of your life.

STEP 4

Talk to Others

Find one or two friends you can talk to about what is going on, preferably friends who are good listeners. If you have friends who are problem solvers, thank them for their ideas but ask them gently if they would mind if you just talk. People like to help and often want to offer solutions or helpful suggestions. These people are well-intentioned. They sometimes just need a reminder that you have things under control.

Consider talking to a therapist, not for purposes of a long-term relationship but just for now. You need all the support you can get right now and a trained professional can help. You can always talk to the hospital's religious professional or social worker, but keep in mind that your needs may exceed their capacity. They might know of a therapist who has dealt with your particular situation before. If you need referrals, ask the primary nurse, religious professional, or social worker.

You can also ask your family doctor for a referral, or ask the doctor in charge of your loved one's case.

STEP 5

Seek Out Other Families

The benefit from finding other families in your situation, either in the waiting room or around the hospital, is a built-in support system and source for information resources. While you are sitting in the waiting room, speak to other family members who might also be waiting.

If you see them regularly, suggest going for coffee in the cafeteria.

> *Find other patients and families who are in the same medical situation. Doctors may be able to refer you to other families.*
>
> DR. DAVID WELLISCH, PHD, CHIEF PSYCHOLOGIST, ADULT DIVISION, DAVID GEFFEN SCHOOL OF MEDICINE, UCLA, LOS ANGELES, CA

Many family members reported that interacting with other family members with loved ones on the same floor was extremely helpful. Not only did it provide comfort, but the exchange of information was also beneficial.

STEP 6

Keep Family and Friends Updated

Keeping family and friends in the loop about the progress of your loved one is a good way to enlist their support. Sometimes, if some time goes by, people tend to forget. They aren't purposely forgetting about you or your loved one, but they get on with their lives and their focus shifts. If you keep them updated with a bi-weekly or weekly email or phone call, you are reminding them that you and your loved one are still coping with the current situation.

Some family members said they changed the message on their answering machine daily to update callers.

STEP 7

Avoid Getting Isolated

It's easy to get isolated when your loved one has been in the hospital for more than a few days. The loneliness that can accompany isolation compounds the problem.

Find an Internet chat room that has people like you who are sharing their experiences about loved ones with the same disease, illness, or injury. If you can't find one, ask the primary nurse, hospital social worker, nurse supervisor, or religious professional if they know of one.

Talk to other family members you see in the hospital. If you're in the waiting room, use the opportunity to find out about them and their loved one. They will in turn, hopefully, ask about you and yours. Ask them if they know of any resources such as chat rooms or in-person support groups.

Family's Story

Steve, whose wife was in the hospital for liver cancer, said this: "I developed a very strong kinship with other families who were visiting loved ones." He expressed appreciation for the support from the family members he met there and felt they were very helpful in offering resources.

If you have a religious affiliation, call your church or synagogue and ask if a religious professional can visit with you and/or the patient. Also ask if it has any support groups for people in your situation. If it doesn't, ask where you might find one.

STEP 8

Research Information on Your Loved One's Illness or Injury

Researching information on your loved one's illness, injury, or disease helps in many ways. It educates you so you can have effective conversations with the doctors and nurses. It also helps you feel more in control so you aren't simply waiting around for information from the doctors and nurses. It also reduces a sense of helplessness.

If you search the Internet, please be aware that not all sites are credible. Sometimes Internet sites are filled with scary information and reports from people who have had bad experiences.

Use the Internet sites in this book (see Appendix) or ask the primary nurse, the media relations person at the hospital, a hospital administrator, nurse supervisor, or charge nurse for credible websites to do research on your loved one's disease, illness, or injury. Don't forget to record the pertinent information on the Research page in the Quick Reference Guide.

Notes

Notes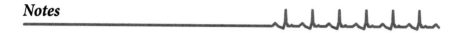

CHAPTER 17

Discharge Planning and Aftercare

Discharge planning starts upon admission.

ALLYSON, RN, SAN FRANCISCO, CA

HOSPITALS ACROSS THE COUNTRY are cutting all or parts of their discharge planning departments. This doesn't mean there won't be help in preparing for your loved one's discharge from the hospital, but there may be less help. To be prepared for discharge, follow these steps:

STEP 1

Ask Questions About Your Role

Most nurses said you should be present at the time of discharge. If the patient is returning home, you'll want to know what kind of care will be needed. Make a list of questions before the time of discharge. Write down the answers in the Quick Reference Guide, page 170. You will refer to these notes later.

Put together a list for what the patient needs. Ask questions about patient care before they leave the hospital. Especially now, with patients being discharged prematurely. Ask the primary nurse for further instructions for discharge if you aren't getting enough answers from the discharge planning department.

ANGIE, RN, PHILADELPHIA, PA

137

Ask the primary nurse to go over all daily care of the patient. Ask the nurse to show you what the patient needs on any given day. Watching someone complete tasks is helpful, rather than relying only on your written notes.

STEP 2

List Doctor Visits

Ask which doctor to call if something goes wrong or if the patient isn't recovering well at home. Write down, in the Discharge and Post-discharge Care section, the name and phone numbers of the doctor you are to call.

Be sure to write down when the patient is to see which doctors. This is very important. The doctors may not follow up with you about future scheduled appointments with the patient. You need to ask. Write it down.

STEP 3

List Medications

Get a list of medications your loved one is to take after they are back home. Rachel, an RN from Chicago, IL, suggested getting prescriptions filled before the patient goes home. List the medications on page 170.

STEP 4

List Diet Restrictions

Ask the primary nurse, discharge planner, or case manager if there are any dietary restrictions for the patient. If so, write them on page 170.

STEP 5

Find Out Who Will Help You

Find out from the primary nurse, discharge planner, or case manager which professionals will be coming to your home to help out with the patient's needs. Write down their titles, names if you can get them, and whom to call if they don't show up.

Ask the primary nurse, discharge planner, or case manager if you will need to hire a private duty nurse to help with home care. Get a list of references. Write them down.

Ask if your loved one will need someone to be with them at all times.

STEP 6

Ask About the Patient's Recovery

Ask the primary nurse, discharge planner, or case manager what the anticipated recovery time will be. Record the information they give you in this book.

STEP 7

What to Do if the Patient is to Be Discharged Early

Insurance companies try to be the decision makers about when a patient is to be discharged. If you feel your loved one is being discharged too early, bring it up with the primary nurse, the doctor, and if necessary, the charge nurse and nurse supervisor. Explain your concerns. Use your progress notes in this book to support your belief.

Remember:
Your input can effect a
positive change.

Family's Story

Shelly's mother, Mona, was discharged from the hospital and was transferred to a nursing home with rehab facilities. Before the transfer, Shelly had looked at two nursing homes, and one appeared more cheerful. She liked the manager.

Her mother stayed in this facility for one month. In that one month, Mona, who had diabetes, was not given the proper diet, was left confined to her bed on a consistent basis, and was left in a diaper and developed a rash. Shelly also was told by her mom that one night a nurse and technician were kissing in her room when they thought she was asleep.

Now, you can't prevent all these situations from occurring, but there are things you can do. You can research the ratings on nursing homes and rehab facilities, and check to see if there have been any disciplinary actions. You can show up at times when you're not expected, such as afternoons or mornings.

STEP 8

Research Rehab Facilities, Nursing Homes, and Assisted Living Facilities

If your loved one is to be transferred to one of these facilities after being discharged from the hospital, you have a choice as to which one your loved one goes to. Your insurance company probably has more say than you do, but you need to sit down with the case manager and sift through the options.

With both my mother and godmother, I researched a number of rehab facilities and nursing homes. I visited three and four respectively. They are required to have a state-mandated document that shows whether there have been any disciplinary actions, and they are legally bound to show it to you. I asked each one to see theirs.

Go look at two or three of these facilities that are available to your loved one. Talk to the manager there. Talk to the nurses. Ask what percentage of the residents are rehab and what percentage are long-term care. If your loved one is expected to be there for a week, ask yourself if you want them in a place that is 90% long-term care residents. Maybe not.

A facility with a greater percentage of rehab residents is a better place for a patient who is going to be discharged at some point. If your loved one is in need of long-term care, visit at least three facilities and use your gut instincts. Ask to see their documents on disciplinary actions.

Use the Internet. Google "nursing home ratings." Go to www.healthgrades.com to research nursing homes.

Ask each place how much physical therapy, occupational therapy, and how many activities are provided for the patient. Ask if the nurses there are registered nurses or at least LVNs. Ask if there is a social worker on staff.

Once you've done the homework, the best next step is to use your instincts. Is it a happy place? Are the patients well taken care of? Plan to visit your loved one often and observe the quality of care at the facility.

Notes

Quick Reference Guide

Patient's Personal Information

Patient name

Patient's contact information

Name of hospital patient is in

Name of hospital floor	**Patient's hospital room direct phone line**

Date patient admitted to hospital

Patient insurance information

Point person (main person who represents the patient—name and contact information)

Family members' and close friends' contact information

Patient's Medical Information

Current medications

Over-the-counter medications, supplements, herbs, and vitamins

---

Allergies to medications

Other allergies (food, flowers, etc.)

Current symptoms, illnesses, and medical conditions

Past symptoms, illnesses, and surgeries

Patient's Medical Information, cont.

Patient's baseline vital signs (Write down patient's baseline vital signs. Follow up only with changes or abnormalities in vital signs. Note these in the Daily Progress Notes section.)

Date	Blood pressure	Oxygen level	Pulse	Temperature	Other

Patient diagnosis

Doctor who made diagnosis

Treatment plan

Doctor who created treatment plan

Patient's Medical Information, cont.

New medications and dosages

Patient prognosis

Expected length of stay for the patient

Planned surgery, date

Pre-op appointment, date

Possible referrals for a second opinion

Patient's Medical Information, cont.

Notes on conversations with primary physicians (list date)

Notes on conversations with primary nurses (list date)

Notes on conversations with other physicians (list date)

Sample Questions for Doctors and Primary Nurses

1. What is the diagnosis of the patient's illness/injury? Can you please explain that to me?

2. My loved one has (name) disease/injury. Can you please explain the treatment to me? Are there any risks? Does the patient understand those risks?

3. Is my loved one on any new medications or IV fluids/medications? What are those for? Is the patient on the same medications as from home? If not, why not?

4. What are the planned procedures for the patient? Can you explain what those are exactly?

5. Other questions:

Physicians/Nurses/Specialists

Patient's family physician (contact information: phone, cell phone, email)

Patient's primary physician (contact information: phone, cell phone, email)

Patient's specialists (such as pulmonologist, cardiologist; names and contact information)

Primary nurses (names, contact information)

Day shift

Night shift

Day shift

Night shift

Day shift

Night shift

Family Advocate Team

Point person (name and contact information)

Family Advocate Team members (names and contact information)

Private duty nurse, sitter, or companion (names and contact information)

Friends to approach to sit with patient (names and contact information)

Families who could share private duty nurses (names and contact information)

Medication Information

Medication Name	Dosage	Description	Date

Oxygen, TPN, Monitors, IV

Oxygen	Date

TPN	Date

Monitors	Date

IV	Date

Lab and Test Results

Lab Results	Date

Test Results	Date

Procedures and Treatments

Procedure or Treatment	Date

Errors and/or Problems

Date	Medical Professionals Involved	Description of Events

Errors and/or Problems, cont.

Conversations about errors with physician, primary nurse, nurse supervisor (list dates)

Social Worker Information

Social worker's name, office location in hospital, contact information

Social worker's hours and days in hospital

Resources provided by social worker

Whom to contact if there is no hospital social worker

What I Can Do to Help with Patient Care

What I can do to help the nurses

Food I can bring in for the patient

Things I can bring from home

☐ Pajamas   ☐ Additional items

☐ Shampoo, hairbrush, razor

☐ Meals (what is allowed?)

☐ Photos

☐ Get well cards

☐ Newspapers, magazines, books, books on tape

☐ Tape recorder and headphones

☐ CD player and headphones

☐ MP3 player

☐ DVD player and headphones

☐ Blanket

Assisting the Patient

Whom can I contact for spiritual help for the patient? (Names and phone numbers)

Do I need to call the patient's employer? (name and phone number)

Are there pets at the patient's home? If so, what arrangements will I make for the pets?

Friends and family the patient wants me to contact about his/her hospitalization (names and phone numbers)

Fall Prevention Information

Patient confined to bed, date

_____

Fall risk?

_____

Assigned sitter, companion, or private duty nurse

_____

Patient's Dietary Restrictions

_____

Cultural Preferences and Issues

_____

Patient's New Hospital Floor

Date

Patient's new room number	Patient's direct phone number

Primary nurses (contact information)

Day shift

Night shift

New medications

New dietary restrictions

Research on Patient's Illness/Injury

Hospital library resources

Internet websites recommended by doctors and nurses

Resources recommended by other patients' families

Possible alternative treatments

If You Live Out of Town

Housing and hotels

Transportation

Local family members and friends

Hospital social worker

Private duty nurses, sitters, and companions

Further questions to ask

Notes

Considering a Different Hospital

New hospital under consideration

Name _____

Location_____

Contact information _____

_____

Is the patient stabilized?

Is a move recommended by the patient's primary physician?

Research on the new hospital

Health Directive Documents

☐ Advance Directive

☐ Living Will

☐ Durable Power of Attorney for Health Care

☐ DNR

Notes

Taking Care of You

Religious professional, contact phone number

Support groups

Taking Care of You, cont.

Other families

Therapists

Chat rooms

Taking Care of You, cont.

Friends I can talk to

People I can call for help

Hospital social worker, contact phone number

Websites

Other things I can do for me

Discharge and Post-Discharge Care

Doctor visits (who and when)

List of medications

Diet

Discharge and Post-Discharge Care, cont.

Notes for daily home care of the patient

Private duty nurses (names and contact information)

Discharge and Post-Discharge Care, cont.

Nurses and therapists (OT, PT, etc.) who will visit (names and contact information)

Anticipated time for recovery

Rehab facilities, assisted living facilities, and nursing homes

Notes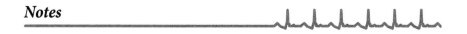

Notes

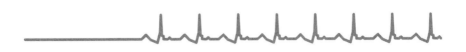

Daily Progress Notes

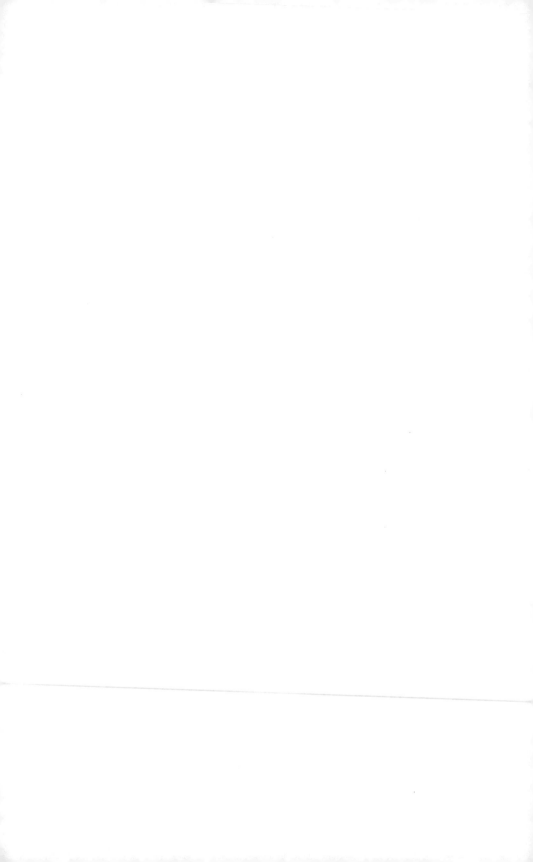

Daily Progress Notes—Day 1

Date

Point person and/or team member schedule (who shows up and when)

Name	Date	Time

What is planned for today? (Procedures, treatments, or surgeries)

Daily Progress Notes—Day 1, cont.

Questions for doctors

Notes on meeting with primary physician

Notes on meeting with specialists or other physicians

Daily Progress Notes—Day 1, cont.

Questions for primary nurses

Notes on meeting with primary nurses

Daily conversations with nurses and doctors

Possible referrals for a second opinion (if necessary)

Changes in patient's medications (List new medications/IV and dosages.)

Daily Progress Notes—Day 1, cont.

Patient observations (Note how the patient is doing physically and emotionally, changes in vital signs, changes in lab or test results. Only note what is unusual or abnormal. Compare to the patient's baseline.)

General notes

Daily Progress Notes—Day 2

Date

Point person and/or team member schedule (who shows up and when)

Name	Date	Time

What is planned for today? (Procedures, treatments, or surgeries)

Daily Progress Notes—Day 2, cont.

Questions for doctors

Notes on meeting with primary physician

Notes on meeting with specialists or other physicians

Daily Progress Notes—Day 2, cont.

Questions for primary nurses

Notes on meeting with primary nurses

Daily conversations with nurses and doctors

Possible referrals for a second opinion (if necessary)

Changes in patient's medications (List new medications/IV and dosages.)

Daily Progress Notes—Day 2, cont.

Patient observations (Note how the patient is doing physically and emotionally, changes in vital signs, changes in lab or test results. Only note what is unusual or abnormal. Compare to the patient's baseline.)

General notes

Daily Progress Notes—Day 3

Date

Point person and/or team member schedule (who shows up and when)

Name	Date	Time

What is planned for today? (Procedures, treatments, or surgeries)

Daily Progress Notes—Day 3, cont.

Questions for doctors

Notes on meeting with primary physician

Notes on meeting with specialists or other physicians

Daily Progress Notes—Day 3, cont.

Questions for primary nurses

Notes on meeting with primary nurses

Daily conversations with nurses and doctors

Possible referrals for a second opinion (if necessary)

Changes in patient's medications (List new medications/IV and dosages.)

Daily Progress Notes—Day 3, cont.

Patient observations (Note how the patient is doing physically and emotionally, changes in vital signs, changes in lab or test results. Only note what is unusual or abnormal. Compare to the patient's baseline.)

General notes

Daily Progress Notes—Day 4

Date

Point person and/or team member schedule (who shows up and when)

Name	Date	Time

What is planned for today? (Procedures, treatments, or surgeries)

Daily Progress Notes—Day 4, cont.

Questions for doctors

Notes on meeting with primary physician

Notes on meeting with specialists or other physicians

Daily Progress Notes—Day 4, cont.

Questions for primary nurses

Notes on meeting with primary nurses

Daily conversations with nurses and doctors

Possible referrals for a second opinion (if necessary)

Changes in patient's medications (List new medications/IV and dosages.)

Daily Progress Notes—Day 4, cont.

Patient observations (Note how the patient is doing physically and emotionally, changes in vital signs, changes in lab or test results. Only note what is unusual or abnormal. Compare to the patient's baseline.)

General notes

Daily Progress Notes—Day 5

Date

Point person and/or team member schedule (who shows up and when)

Name	Date	Time

What is planned for today? (Procedures, treatments, or surgeries)

Daily Progress Notes—Day 5, cont.

Questions for doctors

Notes on meeting with primary physician

Notes on meeting with specialists or other physicians

Daily Progress Notes—Day 5, cont.

Questions for primary nurses

Notes on meeting with primary nurses

Daily conversations with nurses and doctors

Possible referrals for a second opinion (if necessary)

Changes in patient's medications (List new medications/IV and dosages.)

Daily Progress Notes—Day 5, cont.

Patient observations (Note how the patient is doing physically and emotionally, changes in vital signs, changes in lab or test results. Only note what is unusual or abnormal. Compare to the patient's baseline.)

General notes

Daily Progress Notes—Day 6

Date

Point person and/or team member schedule (who shows up and when)

Name	Date	Time

What is planned for today? (Procedures, treatments, or surgeries)

Daily Progress Notes—Day 6, cont.

Questions for doctors

Notes on meeting with primary physician

Notes on meeting with specialists or other physicians

Daily Progress Notes—Day 6, cont.

Questions for primary nurses

Notes on meeting with primary nurses

Daily conversations with nurses and doctors

Possible referrals for a second opinion (if necessary)

Changes in patient's medications (List new medications/IV and dosages.)

Daily Progress Notes—Day 6, cont.

Patient observations (Note how the patient is doing physically and emotionally, changes in vital signs, changes in lab or test results. Only note what is unusual or abnormal. Compare to the patient's baseline.)

General notes

Daily Progress Notes—Day 7

Date

Point person and/or team member schedule (who shows up and when)

Name	Date	Time

What is planned for today? (Procedures, treatments, or surgeries)

Daily Progress Notes—Day 7, cont.

Questions for doctors

Notes on meeting with primary physician

Notes on meeting with specialists or other physicians

Daily Progress Notes—Day 7, cont.

Questions for primary nurses

Notes on meeting with primary nurses

Daily conversations with nurses and doctors

Possible referrals for a second opinion (if necessary)

Changes in patient's medications (List new medications/IV and dosages.)

Daily Progress Notes—Day 7, cont.

Patient observations (Note how the patient is doing physically and emotionally, changes in vital signs, changes in lab or test results. Only note what is unusual or abnormal. Compare to the patient's baseline.)

General notes

Hospital Staff Glossary

Doctors

Anesthesiologist: administers medicine during surgery to help the patient fall asleep.

Attending Physician: leads the health care team in a teaching hospital and has overall responsibility for the patient's care. Along with the Resident doctor, the Attending doctor examines the patient, monitors daily progress, plans care, and oversees treatment.

Cardiologist: doctor who specializes in treating heart or blood vessel problems.

Consulting Physician: doctor who has an area of expertise and may be asked to help diagnose and treat the patient. Can be brought in for a consultation by the primary care physician.

Endocrinologist: doctor who specializes in treating diseases and conditions caused by hormone problems. An endocrinologist also treats diabetes and certain metabolic problems.

Fellow: licensed doctor in a teaching hospital who has completed his/her residency program and is completing additional advanced training in another specialty area.

Gastroenterologist: doctor who specializes in digestive diseases.

Hematologist: doctor who specializes in the functions and disorders of the blood.

Hepatologist: doctor who specializes in liver diseases.

Hospitalist: hospital doctor who cares for all hospital patients.

Intensivist: hospital doctor assigned to take care of all critical care patients in the hospital.

Nephrologist: doctor who specializes in the kidneys.

Neurologist: doctor who specializes in the brain and spinal chord.

OB/GYN: doctor who specializes in obstetrics and gynecology.

Oncologist: doctor who specializes in treating cancer.

Orthopedist: doctor who diagnoses, treats, manages the rehabilitation process, and provides prevention protocols for patients who suffer from injury or disease in any part of the musculoskeletal system.

Physician Assistant: health professional licensed to practice medicine with doctor supervision. He/she makes medical decisions and provides a broad range of diagnostic therapeutic services.

Primary Care Physician: doctor who provides patients with a broad spectrum of health care, both preventive and curative, and coordinates all the care patients require, including referral to specialist physicians.

Pulmonologist: doctor who specializes in treating lung problems.

Radiologist: doctor who specializes in radiology.

Resident: licensed doctor in a teaching hospital who is receiving additional specialty training. During his/her residency program, he/she provides care under the supervision of the Attending doctor.

Specialist: doctor who has advanced training and experience in identifying and treating diseases and conditions of particular parts of the body. For example, a cardiologist treats conditions related to the heart.

Surgeon: doctor who operates on the patient if they are having surgery.

Nurses

Registered Nurse (RN): nurse who has graduated from a formal program of nursing education and is licensed by the state. They are responsible for all general nursing care and for teaching patients and their families. Also called the primary nurse.

Charge Nurse/Nurse Manager: supervisor who is assigned the responsibility of supervising the nurses during a particular shift. He/she can help solve problems for families and patients.

Nurse Practitioner: registered nurse with a master's degree and training in the diagnosis and management of common and complex medical conditions. Many NPs serve as mid-level primary health care providers. In some states, NPs admit and follow their patients through their hospitalizations.

Clinical Nurse Specialist: advanced practice RN who functions as a health provider, educator, consultant, researcher, administrator or case manager. The CNS usually has a specialty practice and has had several years of practice in a clinical nursing specialty. He/she has a masters or doctoral degree.

LVN or LPN: licensed vocational nurse, or licensed practical nurse who is under supervision of the primary nurse or doctor. Most can take blood pressure and draw blood but also do bathing of the patient and clean up.

CNA or Nursing Assistant/Aide: supervised by the primary nurse, he/she helps with patient care. His/her duties can include taking blood pressure, pulse, bathing, serving meals, assisting the patient to walk or get out of bed, turning the patient in bed, and clean up. Can oversee patient safety.

Therapists and Technicians

Occupational Therapist (OT): provides assessment and therapy to patients facing challenges with motor, sensory, cognitive perceptual, and psychosocial development. They help patients gain maximum independence in their daily life.

Phlebotomist (or IV Team): draws blood from the patient for various medical tests. This could also be performed by a nurse.

Physical Therapist (PT): helps patients regain muscle strength through specially designed exercises.

Respiratory Therapist: provides care to patients who have difficulty breathing.

Social Worker: licensed counselor who helps patients and families with emotional, physical, and financial problems related to the patient's illness. He/she is available to help during hospitalization and discharge. He/she also helps patients and families connect with needed community resources.

Speech Therapist: works with patients who have difficulty talking or making certain sounds.

Medical Terms Glossary

O₂: Oxygen.

A Fib: atrial fibrillation. Fluttering of the upper chamber of the heart.

Abscess: collection of pus caused by local infection.

Acute: refers to a medical problem that needs immediate attention. Can also refer to severe, sharp pain.

Advance Directive: document written in advance of serious illness that states your loved one's choices for health care, or names someone to make those choices if your loved one becomes unable to.

AMI: acute myocardial infarction. Heart attack.

Analgesic: any drug intended to relieve pain.

Anaphylactic shock: intense allergic reaction to a substance such as a drug or venom that leads to difficulty in breathing and speaking, low blood pressure, rapid pulse, sweating, and collapse.

Angiogram: x-ray of the arteries and veins to detect blockage or narrowing of vessels.

Angioplasty: use of a small balloon on the tip of a catheter that is inserted into a blood vessel to open up an area of blockage inside the vessel.

Arrhythmia: variation in the regular rhythm of the heartbeat.

Aspiration: removal of a sample of fluid and cells through a needle.

Barium: metallic, chemical, chalky liquid to coat the inside of the organs so they will show up on an x-ray.

Bedsores: ulcers that occur on areas of the skin that are under pressure from lying in bed, sitting in wheelchairs, wearing a cast, or being immobile for a long period of time.

Benign: term to describe a tumor that is noncancerous.

BID: twice a day, or every 12 hours.

Blood count: number of red blood cells, white blood cells, and platelets in a sample of blood. Also referred to as CBC.

Blood pressure (BP): measure of the force of blood flow against veins and arteries.

Cardiac: pertaining to the heart.

Cardiac arrest: heart stops beating.

Catheter: thin, flexible tube that carries fluids in or out of the body.

CBC: complete blood count.

Central line: intravenous line inserted into a large vein in the neck.

Chronic: refers to a disease or disorder that usually develops slowly and lasts for a long period of time.

CNS: central nervous system.

CPAP: continuous airway pressure by a ventilator to keep the airways open.

CPR: cardio-pulmonary resuscitation.

CT or CAT scan: three-dimensional image of an internal part of the body, constructed by computer from a cross-section of images. CT scans reveal internal organs, bone, soft tissues, and blood vessels. More detailed than x-rays.

Defibrillator: electronic device used to establish normal heartbeat.

Dialysis: medical procedure to remove wastes and additional fluid from the blood after the kidneys have stopped functioning.

DNR: do not resuscitate

ECG or EKG (electrocardiogram): graphic record of the action of the heart.

Echocardiogram: ultrasound test that uses sound waves to examine the heart in motion.

Edema: abnormal buildup of fluid that causes swelling.

EEG (electroencephalogram): measures electrical activity in the brain.

Embolism: blockage of a blood vessel, such as a blood clot.

ER: emergency room.

Gastro: refers to stomach or abdomen.

Gastrostomy tube: surgically placed tube that goes directly into the stomach for feedings and/or drainage.

General anesthetic: anesthetic that causes the patient to become unconscious during surgery.

GI series: tests of the digestive system.

Hematoma: swelling that contains blood, usually clotted, in an organ, space, or tissue.

Hemorrhage: excessive bleeding.

Hepatic: related to the liver.

Hyperglycemia: abnormally high blood-sugar level. (Hypo means low.)

Hypertension: abnormally high blood pressure. (Hypo means low.)

ICU: intensive care unit.

Imaging: tests or evaluation procedures that produce pictures of areas inside the body.

Informed consent: legal document that explains the course of treatment, the risks, the benefits, and possible alternatives. The process by which a patient agrees to treatment.

Intubate: to place a breathing tube down the throat of a patient who requires breathing assistance.

Intubation: insertion of a tube into a hollow organ, such as the trachea.

IV: intravenous. The delivery of fluids and/or medication into the blood stream via a needle inserted into a vein.

Laparoscopy: test that uses a tube with a light and camera lens to examine internal organs and to check for abnormalities. Laparoscopy is often used during surgery to look inside the body and to avoid making a large incision.

Living Will: legal document that states your medical preferences for treatment and resuscitation in the event you can no longer speak for yourself.

Malignant: dangerous to health.

MI: myocardial infarction, heart attack.

Monitor: visual screen that exhibits the patient's vital statistics.

MRI (magnetic resonance imaging): computerized images that provide 3-D images of the body's interior, which shows muscle, bone, blood vessels, nerves, organs, and tumor tissue.

MRSA: methicillin-resistant staphylococcus aureus.

Nasal cannula: plastic tube with two prongs that are placed in the nose to deliver oxygen to the patient.

Nastrogastric tube (NG tube): tube that leads from the nose or mouth into the stomach.

Nosocomial: infection acquired in the hospital.

NPO: nothing by mouth; nothing to eat or drink, usually within a defined time frame.

Nuclear medicine: specialized area of radiology that uses very small amounts of radioactive substances to examine organ function and structure.

Nurse-to-patient ratio: number of patients that a nurse is responsible for. High ratio means fewer patients to a nurse, and low ratio means higher number of patients per nurse.

Open heart surgery: surgery that involves opening the chest and heart, while a heart-lung machine performs for the heart.

OR: operating room.

Pain threshold: least amount of pain a patient can recognize.

Pain tolerance level: most pain a patient can tolerate.

Palliative: relieving the symptoms or pain of a disease or disorder without affecting the cure.

Palpitation: condition when the heart pounds or races.

PET scan: positron emission tomography. A type of nuclear medicine imaging.

PICC line: peripherally inserted central catheter for delivery of medication into bloodstream.

PIC-U: pediatric intensive care unit.

Pneumonia: serious inflammation or infection of one or both lungs. Thickening of the fluids in lungs can be associated.

Port: semi-permanent opening of a vein for use with IV therapy.

Post-op: post-operative.

Power of Attorney (power of attorney for health care): specifies a specific person to legally make a decision for a patient who isn't able to do this for him or herself.

Pre-op: pre-operative.

PRN: when necessary; on request or when needed within time guidelines.

Prognosis: likely course of a disease or condition.

QD: once a day.

Qh: every hour.

QID: four times daily.

QOD: every other day.

Radiology: x-rays and other imaging techniques.

RBC: red blood cells.

Rehab: rehabilitation.

Renal failure: inability of the body's kidneys to function.

Respirator (ventilator): apparatus to administer artificial respiration (used when a patient cannot breathe on their own).

Respiratory failure: acute or chronic condition in which the function of the lungs is markedly impaired.

Rounds: doctors' visitation to the patients.

Sepsis: bacterial infection in the blood.

SNF: skilled nursing facility.

Spinal tap (lumbar puncture): procedure to isolate cerebral spinal fluid for evaluation or diagnosis.

Stat: immediately, urgent.

Stent: tiny, expandable coil that is placed inside a blood vessel at the site of blockage. The stent is expanded to open the blockage.

Step-Down Unit: hospital floor below ICU and above other floors.

Stroke: happens when the brain cells die because of inadequate blood flow to the brain.

Subcutaneous: under the skin.

Tachycardia: rapid heart beat.

Thrombosis: excess clotting which obstructs veins and arteries.

TID: three times a day.

Titrate: to gradually increase the dose of a drug.

TPN: total parenteral nutrition. Feeding a person intravenously.

TPR: temperature, pulse, respirations.

Trach: abbreviation for tracheostomy tube.

Tracheostomy: surgical procedure to create an opening in the neck into the trachea.

Tracheotomy: cutting an airway into the trachea.

Triage: section of the hospital where personnel question the newly admitted patient to assign placement.

Ultrasound: diagnostic imaging technique that uses high frequency sound waves and a computer to create images of blood vessels, tissues, and organs.

V Fib: ventricular fibrillation. Contraction of the heart's ventricles.

Vascular: pertaining to blood vessels.

Ventilator: machine that regularly pumps air in and out of the lungs when normal breathing isn't possible.

Vital signs: heart rate and rhythm, blood pressure, and respiration.

WBC: measure of white blood cells.

X-ray: type of radiation used for imaging purposes to provide a picture.

References

ABC News. "Deadly Hospital Infections Occurring More." Primetime, October 23, 2003. http://abcnews.go.com/Primetime/story?id=132442&page=1

ABC World News Tonight. "Nursing Shortage: How It May Affect You." January 21, 2006. http://abcnews.go.com/WNT/Health/story?id=1529546

American Hospital Association. *The State of America's Hospitals—Taking the Pulse. Findings from the AHA 2006 Survey of Hospital Leaders.* American Hospital Association.http://www.aha.org/aha/content/2006/PowerPoint/StateHospitalsChartPack2006.PPT

Beers, Mark H., ed. *Merck Manual of Medical Information.* 2d home ed. New York: Random House, 1997.

CBS News. "Nursing Shortage in Critical Stage." 60 Minutes, January 17, 2003. http://www.cbsnews.com/stories/2003/01/17/60minutes/main536999.shtml

Clayman, Charles B., medical ed. *The American Medical Association Family Medical Guide.* 3d ed. New York: Random House, 1995.
Fox, Maggie, Health and Science Correspondent for Reuters. "Complex ICU situations cause deadly errors: report."(February 15, 2006). http://www.redorbit.com/news/health/391323/complex_icu_situations_cause_deadly_errors_report/

Gibbs, Nancy, and Amanda Bauer. "Q: What Scares Doctors? A: Being the Patient." *Time,* May 1, 2006. http://www.time.com/time/magazine/article/0,9171,1186553,00.html

Greider, Katharine. "Dirty Hospitals: Two million patients are infected in hospitals each year and 90,000 of those Americans die." *AARP Bulletin,* January 2007. http://www.hospitalinfection.org/press/010107aarp.doc

Health Grades. *HealthGrades Quality Study: Third Annual Patient Safety in American Hospitals Study.* Health Grades, Inc., April 2006. http://www.healthgrades.com/media/DMS/pdf /PatientSafetyInAmericanHospitalsStudy2006.pdf

Health Grades. *The Fifth Annual HealthGrades Patient Safety in American Hospitals Study.* Health Grades, Inc., April 2008. http://www. healthgrades.com/media/DMS/pdf /PatientSafetyInAmericanHospitalsStudy2008.pdf

Institute of Medicine of the National Academies. *Preventing Medication Errors.* Report Brief. Institute of Medicine of the National Academies, July 2006. http://www.iom.edu/Object.File/Master/35/943 /medication errors new.pdf

Klevens, R. Monina, Jonathan R. Edwards, Chesley L. Richards, Jr., Teresa C. Horan, Robert P. Gaynes, Daniel A. Pollock, and Denise M. Cardo. "Estimating Health Care-Associated Infections and Deaths in U.S. Hospitals, 2002." *Public Health Reports* 122 (March-April 2007): 160-166. Centers for Disease Control and Prevention. http://www.cdc .gov/ncidod/dhqp/pdf/hicpac/infections_deaths.pdf

Marquez, Laura. "Nursing Shortage: How It May Affect You." ABC News, Jan. 21, 2006. http://abcnews.go.com/WNT/Health/story?id=1529546

National Institute of Allergy and Infectious Diseases. *The Problem of Antimicrobial Resistance.* National Institute of Allergy and Infectious Diseases, Division of Microbiology and Infectious Diseases. National Institutes of Health, US Department of Health and Human Services, April 2006. http://www.niaid.nih.gov/factsheets/antimicro.htm

Needleman, Jack, Peter Buerhaus, Soeren Mattke, Maureen Stewart, and Katya Zelevinsky. "Nurse-Staffing Levels and the Quality of Care in Hospitals." *New England Journal of Medicine* 346 (May 30, 2002): 1715-1722. http://content.nejm.org/cgi/content/abstract/346/22/1715

Santell, John P. "Medication Errors in Intensive Care Units." *US Pharm.* 2006 (5): 56-59. http://www.uspharmacist.com/index .asp?show=article&page=8_1738.htm

Underwood, Anne. "Diagnosis: Not Enough Nurses." *Newsweek,* December 12, 2005. http://www.newsweek.com/id/51387

Appendix:
Useful Websites
for Further Research

Common Medical Terms Used in Hospitals

http://www.nyp.org/glossary/index

Illnesses, Medical Conditions, or Injuries

http://www.medlineplus.gov

http://www.merck.com

http://www.webMD.com

http://www.healthfinder.gov

http://www.mayoclinic.com

http://www.cdc.gov

http://www.HHS.gov (Information about health-related resources)

http://www.NIH.gov (National Institute of Health)

Medication Errors and Drug Interactions

U.S. Food and Drug Administration Center for Drug Evaluation
and Research: http://www.fda.gov/CDER/drug/MedErrors
/default.htm

Institute for Safe Medication Practices (They provide medication
safety tools and resources) http://www.ismp.org

Best Hospitals in US

http://health.usnews.com/sections/health/best-hospitals

Patient Safety

http://www.jcipatientsafety.org (The Joint Commission's Center
for Patient Safety)

Family and Patient Support

http://www.carepages.com

Hospitals and Nursing Homes

http://www.healthgrades.com
http://www.nursingworld.org
http://www.jointcommission.org

Index

For More Information

Visit www.criticalconditions.com for further information and updates on how to be an effective advocate for your hospitalized loved one. Included are further resources, recent news on the US health care system, a place for families to share their personal stories about caring for hospitalized loved ones, upcoming events, more information from physicians, nurses and hospital staff, and links to resources.

To Contact the Author

If you wish to contact Martine Ehrenclou or would like more information, please go to info@criticalconditions.com. Every effort will be made to respond to each request.

If you wish to write a letter, please write to Martine Ehrenclou, c/o Lemon Grove Press LLC, 1223 Wilshire Blvd., Suite 1750, Santa Monica, CA 90403-5400.

To Order *Critical Conditions*

Critical Conditions by Martine Ehrenclou, MA, is available through your favorite book dealer or from the publisher:

Lemon Grove Press, LLC
1223 Wilshire Blvd., Suite 1750
Santa Monica, CA 90403-5400

info@criticalconditions.com
www.criticalconditions.com
Fax: (310) 451-1968

Critical Conditions, ISBN-978-0-9815240-0-9, is available for $19.95, plus $5.50 for shipping and handling ($2 for each additional copy), plus sales tax for CA orders.

Special discounts are available on quantity purchases by corporations, associations, and others. For details, contact Lemon Grove Press at the above address.